OECD Health Policy Studies

Health Workforce Policies in OECD Countries

RIGHT JOBS, RIGHT SKILLS, RIGHT PLACES

OECD

BETTER POLICIES FOR BETTER LIVES

Please cite this publication as:
OECD (2016), *Health Workforce Policies in OECD Countries: Right Jobs, Right Skills, Right Places*, OECD Health Policy Studies, OECD Publishing, Paris.
http://dx.doi.org/10.1787/9789264239517-en

ISBN 978-92-64-23950-0 (print)
ISBN 978-92-64-23951-7 (PDF)

Series: OECD Health Policy Studies
ISSN 2074-3181 (print)
ISSN 2074-319X (online)

Photo credits: Cover © vladvm50/Fotolia.com; © vladis.studio/Shutterstock.com; © iStock.com/geopaul; ©Olegbabick-Thinkstock; © Zern Liew/Shutterstock.com; © graphixmania/Shutterstock.com

Corrigenda to OECD publications may be found on line at: *www.oecd.org/about/publishing/corrigenda.htm*.

Foreword

Across the OECD, health outcomes have continued to improve, generation after generation. This would not have been possible without the efforts, skills and dedication of millions of health workers. The role of doctors, nurses and other health professionals in delivering health services to the population, thereby contributing to better health outcomes, stronger economies and more vibrant societies, is undeniable. The health and social sector now accounts for 10% of employment in our economies. As the health and long-term care needs of ageing populations grow in size and complexity, it is not surprising that this share is expected to rise, providing many more job opportunities.

There have never been as many doctors and nurses working in OECD countries as now, but concerns about labour and skill shortages loom large in a number of OECD countries. However, filling vacancies for skilled health workers by recruiting from low-income countries risks undermining the progress these countries are making towards better health services. While people have a fundamental right to move from one country to another, OECD countries need to continue to train enough health workers to avoid "free-riding" on the training efforts of other countries.

The time is ripe for addressing the future of health workers across OECD countries and beyond. In September 2015, the United Nations General Assembly adopted the Sustainable Development Goals (SDGs), calling on all countries to achieve tangible improvements in people's lives, including health, education, employment and gender equality, among many others. The OECD has a strong track record in measuring the performance of health systems, and will support global efforts to attain these goals. Without the solid engagement of health workers around the world, it will not be possible to achieve the ambitious SDG goal of providing access to high-quality of care for the whole population at an affordable cost.

The political momentum to strengthen and re-think health workforce strategies for the benefits of all citizens around the world will intensify through the United Nations Secretary-General Commission on Health Employment and Economic Growth chaired by President François Hollande and President Jacob Zuma, of which I am a vice-Chair together with the Director-General of WHO, Dr Margaret Chan, and the Director-General of ILO, Mr. Guy Ryder. Countries need to co-operate more to ensure that the world gets the strategic investments in the health workforce that are necessary to achieve universal health coverage and high-quality care.

This publication provides a solid evidence base and analyses to support the discussions of this United Nations Secretary-General Commission. Following a period of strong expansion in the training capacity of new doctors and nurses in many OECD countries, and successful efforts to increase retention rates in the medical and nursing professions, the main health workforce priorities in the post-crisis period have changed. Within OECD countries, the most pressing problems are how to ensure the right mix, efficient use and proper geographical distribution of health workers. Only with the right numbers of health workers, equipped with the right skills and providing services in the right places, will it be possible to respond equitably and effectively to the changing health needs of ageing populations.

In parallel, health workers will have to adopt innovative ways of delivering health services, taking advantage of the great opportunities opened up by the digitalisation of our daily lives. There must be changes in the traditional functions and responsibilities of health professionals, and this will require reforms of the education and training systems so that they are equipped with the right skills, and are able to adapt them during the working life to address the future health needs of our societies. Through publications like this one, the OECD provides valuable advice in this area, and remains committed to advancing better health policies for better and healthier lives.

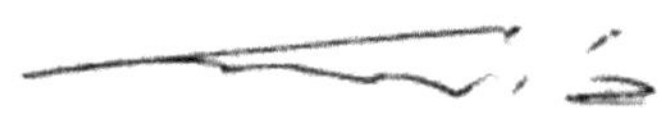

Angel Gurría
OECD Secretary-General

ACKNOWLEDGEMENTS

This publication brings together a series of studies on health workforce issues that were carried out as part of the 2013-14 and 2015-16 programme of work of the OECD Health Committee. It is the culmination of work done over the past few years to gather evidence, analyse and outline policy options to respond to some key health workforce policy priorities identified by the Health Committee.

Several chapters of this publication have benefited from financial support from the European Commission (Chapter 3 on changes in education and training policies and Chapter 6 on skills use and skills mismatch in the health sector) and from the World Health Organization and the Swiss Government (Chapter 4 on the international migration of doctors and nurses). The OECD is grateful to the support that these organisations have provided to this work. The contents of these and other chapters in this publication are the sole responsibility of the OECD and can in no way be taken to reflect the views of the European Union, the World Health Organization or any national government.

The preparation of this report was co-ordinated by Gaétan Lafortune and Liliane Moreira from the OECD Health Division, who also co-authored several chapters. The other authors are (by order of chapters):

- Michael Schoenstein (formerly from the OECD Health Division, now working for the German Federal Ministry of Labour and Social Affairs) who contributed to Chapters 2, 5 and 6.
- Clémence Merçay (formerly from the University of Neuchâtel, now working for the Swiss Health Observatory) who is the lead author on Chapter 4.
- Jean-Christophe Dumont (from the OECD International Migration Division) who contributed to Chapter 4.
- Tomoko Ono (formerly from the OECD Health Division, now working in the health team of the Japan International Cooperation Agency) who contributed to Chapters 5 and 6.
- James Buchan (from Queen Margaret University Edinburgh) who contributed to Chapter 5.

The content of the various chapters benefited from comments and suggestions received by OECD Health Committee delegates and from the data provided by OECD Health Data National Correspondents. Preliminary findings of some chapters also received useful comments during the meetings of the Expert Group on European Health Workforce organised by the European Commission. Francesca Colombo, Mark Pearson and Stefano Scarpetta from the OECD also provided many useful comments and suggestions. Thanks also go to Frédéric Daniel and Gaëlle Balestat for statistical support, and to Emma Pike, Nikolas Kourkoulas and Imane Baïz for valuable research assistance during their internship at the OECD.

Table of contents

Figures

Tables

Executive summary

Health workers are the cornerstone of health systems. Despite all the interest in self-treatment and the growing role of eHealth and mHealth, it is still – overwhelmingly – health workers that provide health services to the population. Jobs in the health and social sector now account for more than 10% of total employment in many OECD countries. In 2013, 3.6 million doctors and 10.8 million nurses were working in OECD countries, up from 2.9 million doctors and 8.3 million nurses in 2000.

Despite this growth, discussions about health workforce issues in OECD countries often continue to focus on shortages of health workers, with persisting concerns that the upcoming retirement of the "baby-boom" generation of doctors and nurses might exacerbate such shortages. This publication finds that OECD countries anticipated this wave of retirement by increasing student intakes in medical and nursing education programmes over the past decade. Many new doctors and nurses are thus expected to enter the labour market to replace those who will retire. In addition, pension reforms and other initiatives have increased retention rates of doctors and nurses in the profession, also contributing to maintain if not increasing the supply. In this context, health workforce concerns have shifted from worries of widespread shortages towards more specific issues related to ensuring the right mix of health workers, with the right skills, and providing services in the right places, to better respond to changing population health needs.

This publication analyses recent trends and policies adopted by OECD countries affecting the demand and supply of health workers. While it focuses on doctors and nurses given the predominant role they continue to play, it also highlights efforts underway to move beyond these traditional professional boundaries. Addressing the future health needs of ageing populations, with many more people living with one or more chronic conditions, will require more innovations in health service delivery than those we have seen so far. There will be a need to use more effectively new technologies and the skills of different categories of health workers at all levels, and to provide more effective access to services to people, wherever they live.

Numerus clausus policies should be supported by more robust information about future job prospects

- *Numerus clausus* policies (the setting of annual quotas on the number of students admitted in different programmes) remain a powerful policy lever for governments to adjust the supply of health workers to projected demand and modify the composition of the health workforce, while keeping budgets under control. But there is a need to make better use of this policy instrument.
- Nearly all OECD countries have decided to increase the number of students admitted to medical and nursing education since 2000 in response to concerns about current or possible future shortages. This will result in growing numbers of

new medical and nursing graduates entering the labour market in the years ahead to replace those who will exit.

- At least one country, Australia, has taken the bold move to abandon its *numerus clausus* policy for nursing and other university programmes (with the notable exception of medical education) to open up entry into higher education. As expected, following the removal of this quota in 2009, the number of students admitted in nursing has increased (by 25% between 2009 and 2013). Interestingly though, it has not increased more rapidly than in the previous years when the *numerus clausus* was still in place (a 40% increase between 2005 and 2009), because of constraints on training capacity and lack of suitable applicants.
- A critical element for health workforce planning and the decision-making of prospective students is the availability of robust labour market information about future skill needs. It is also important for health workforce planning to use a more comprehensive approach that takes into account possible substitutions between different categories of workers, to avoid training too many workers who might usefully be substituted by others.
- A number of countries, such as England, France and Canada, have deliberately increased the number of post-graduate training places in general medicine to address specific concerns about shortages of general practitioners (GPs), although it has not always been easy to attract a sufficient number of medical graduates to fill these places. Complementary actions are needed to make general medicine a more attractive option for new doctors, including narrowing the gap in pay rates compared with other specialties.
- The United States, Canada and the Netherlands have also increased student intakes in advanced education programmes for nurses, such as nurse practitioner (NPs) programmes, to increase the supply of "mid-level" providers and improve access to primary care. Evaluations show that advanced practice nurses with proper training can improve access to services and deliver the same quality of care as GPs for patients with minor illnesses, those requiring routine follow-up, and others. When advanced practice nurses take on some of the tasks previously performed by doctors, this can help free up the time of doctors and provide these services at a lower cost.

Reducing the reliance on foreign-trained health workers

- The Global Code of Practice on the International Recruitment of Health Personnel, adopted by all WHO members in 2010, encourages countries to improve their health workforce planning and respond to their future needs without relying unduly on the training efforts of other countries, particularly low-income countries suffering from acute shortages.
- In 2013-14, some 460 000 foreign-trained doctors and 570 000 foreign-trained nurses were working in OECD countries, accounting for about 17% of all doctors and 6% of nurses on average. More than one-third of these foreign-trained doctors and nurses were coming from other OECD countries. In many countries, the absolute number of foreign-trained doctors and nurses has increased between 2006 and 2013-14, but their share has come down, as the number of domestically-trained doctors and nurses increased more rapidly.

- The United States is by far the main destination country of foreign-trained health workers in absolute numbers, with more than 200 000 doctors and almost 250 000 nurses trained abroad in 2013. However, the inflows of foreign-trained doctors and nurses moving to the United States have come down from their peak of about ten years ago because of growing numbers of domestic graduates, particularly nurses. The main countries of origin of foreign-trained health professionals working in the United States are India (for doctors) and the Philippines (for nurses), although the new inflows from these two countries have fallen sharply in recent years.
- The United Kingdom is the second main country of destination, with more than 48 000 foreign-trained doctors and 86 000 foreign-trained nurses in 2014. As in the United States, the annual inflows of foreign-trained doctors and nurses moving to the United Kingdom have come down from their peak of about ten years ago because of increasing numbers of domestic graduates. However, the inflows of foreign-trained nurses in the United Kingdom have recently bounced back up due to an unexpected increase in demand from NHS employers which cannot readily be met from domestic sources. The composition of foreign-trained doctors has changed significantly in the United Kingdom, with growing numbers coming from other EU countries, notably Greece, Italy and Romania, rather than from Asia or Africa. Similarly for nurses, the recent rise in the number of foreign-trained nurses has been driven mainly by migration from Spain and Portugal.
- Some new EU countries in Central and Eastern Europe have seen a large increase in the emigration of their doctors and nurses to other EU countries. In many cases, this out-migration started before their accession to the European Union, but it accelerated immediately afterwards because of the reduction in barriers to mobility. This has prompted countries like the Czech Republic, the Slovak Republic, Hungary and Romania to take actions to reduce the "push" factor by improving the pay rates and working conditions of doctors and nurses, despite tight budget constraints.

Using technology and changing scope of practice to address the health needs of populations living in underserved areas

- In all OECD countries, the number of doctors per capita tends to be much lower in rural/remote areas and in deprived urban areas. In countries like France and Canada, the number of doctors per population is at least two times lower in rural regions than in urban regions.
- Countries have used a wide range of policies to try to achieve a better geographic distribution of doctors and provide adequate access for people living in underserved areas, with uneven success. These include policies targeting the selection of medical students coming from these underserved areas (e.g., Japan), to providing various types of financial incentives to attract and retain more doctors in these areas (e.g., Australia, Canada, France). A few countries (e.g., Germany) have used regulations to restrict the freedom of new doctors to set up a practice in areas deemed to be adequately supplied, along with some financial incentives to encourage them to locate in under-served areas. Such a policy mix may be the most effective approach to achieve the desired goal.

- Many countries have also promoted various types of innovations in health service delivery to achieve the goal of providing adequate access to services with fewer doctors on site. These include encouraging transfers of competences from doctors to nurses and other local health professionals, and the development of telemedicine to connect patients and doctors at a remote distance, successfully implemented in Canada, Australia and Finland.

Promoting a better match and more efficient use of the skills of health workers

- There is evidence of a considerable mismatch between the skills of health workers and skills requirements for their job. Based on the 2011-12 PIAAC survey, about 50% of doctors and 40% nurses reported being under-skilled for some of the tasks that they have to perform, while an even greater proportion (70% to 80% of doctors and nurses) reported being over-skilled, suggesting an important waste of human capital.
- Under-skilling calls for two broad types of actions: 1) reforms of curricula of initial education and training programmes to make sure that health workers acquire the new skills needed to perform well in new health service delivery models, including greater teamwork skills; and 2) promoting well-designed continuous professional development programmes to ensure that the skills of doctors and nurses are adapted to new tasks and job requirements.
- Regular re-licensing systems can provide strong incentives for doctors and nurses to continue upgrading their skills throughout their professional life. Out of 31 OECD countries, only 12 had implemented any mandatory continuous professional development policy for doctors linked to regular re-licensing in 2012-13.
- Nurses with an advanced university degree are much more likely to report being over-skilled for the job they do compared to those with a lower degree. The expansion of the scope of practice of these more highly-educated nurses would allow them to use their skills more fully.
- Given the large amount of public resources spent on health workers' education and training, properly designed training programmes, including a greater recognition of on-the-job practical training, and a more efficient use of human resources on the workplace is critical to ensuring a greater return on public investments.

Key findings

Over the past decade, it has become increasingly clear that OECD countries need to adapt their health systems to changing population health needs and the growing burden of chronic diseases and mental health problems, moving to more team-based and patient-centred care models.

The adoption of the Sustainable Development Goals (SDGs) during the United Nations Summit in September 2015 has renewed the political commitment for all countries around the world – be they upper, middle or lower income – to promote healthy lives and well-being for all the population and to achieve universal health coverage. Universal health coverage requires not only that people have adequate financial protection against the cost of health care, but also that there are appropriately skilled health workers to provide them with high-quality services when they need it.

The challenge of addressing health workforce requirements to achieve the goal of universal health coverage is obviously much greater in low-income countries, where there is a lower supply of skilled health workers and greater health care needs. But OECD countries also face the challenge of designing better health workforce strategies to meet the changing needs of ageing populations in a more cost-effective and sustainable way. There is growing recognition that this involves the need to develop more team-based care models that optimise the scope of practice of different health care providers, taking fuller advantage of the new opportunities offered by new technologies.

This publication reviews recent trends in health labour markets and related policies in OECD countries, and challenges countries are facing to better respond to future demand. Are we actually seeing a "health workforce crisis" that many people feared only a few years ago as the "baby-boom" generation of doctors and nurses was starting to retire? To what extent have OECD countries reduced their reliance on foreign-trained doctors and nurses by increasing their own domestic training capacity? What are the most promising policies to address the issue of the uneven geographic distribution of health workers within countries? What do we know about skills use and skills mismatch in the health sector? How do countries try to optimise the skill mix of health workers and their scope of practice?

1. The number of doctors and nurses has never been greater in OECD countries

Despite repeated claims in the media and in public discussions of "growing shortages" or "crisis", the number of doctors and nurses has never been greater in OECD countries, both in absolute number and on a per capita basis. In 2013, a total of 3.6 million doctors and 10.8 million nurses were employed in OECD countries, up from 2.9 million doctors and 8.3 million nurses in 2000. The number of doctors and nurses has grown more rapidly than the overall population in nearly all countries, so the doctor-to-population and nurse-to-population ratios have increased. On average across OECD countries, there were 3.3 doctors per 1 000 population in 2013, up from 2.7 in 2000 (an increase of 20%), and 9.1 nurses per 1 000 population in 2013, up from 7.8 in 2000 (an increase of 15%).

The growth in the number of doctors has been particularly rapid in some countries, such as Turkey, Korea and Mexico, which started with relatively low levels in 2000, thereby narrowing the gap with other OECD countries. The number of doctors has also increased strongly in the United Kingdom, by over 50% in absolute terms, so that the number of doctors per population in the United Kingdom now exceeds the number in the United States and Canada, although it still remains below the (rising) OECD average. The number of doctors has also increased in other OECD countries that already had a relatively large number of doctors in 2000 (such as Greece, Austria and Norway), albeit in some cases at a slower pace following the economic crisis that started in 2008-09 (Figure 1).

Figure 1. Rising numbers of doctors in OECD countries, 2000 and 2013 (or nearest year)

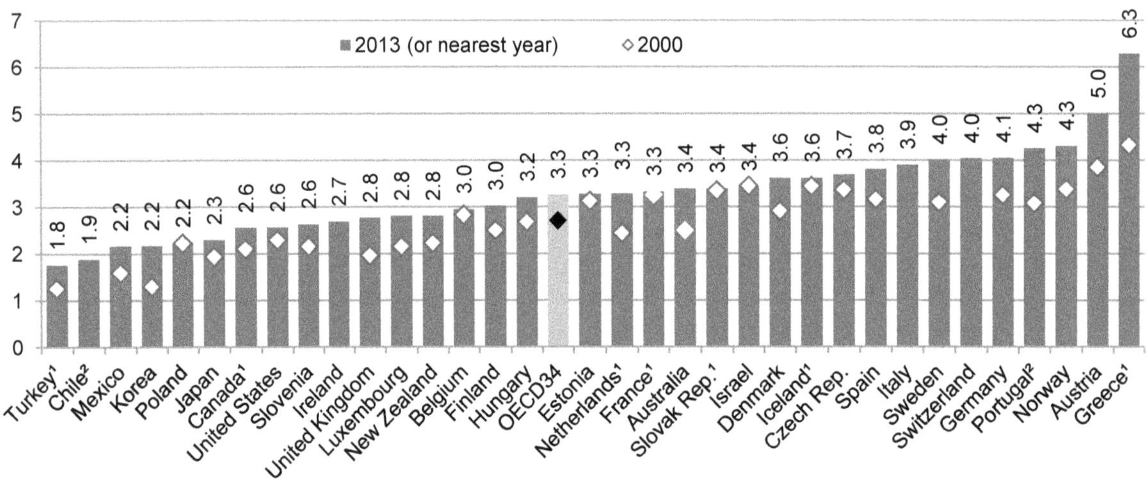

Information on data for Israel: http://dx.doi.org/10.1787/888932315602.

1. Data include not only doctors providing direct care to patients, but also those working in the health sector as managers, educators, researchers, etc. (adding another 5-10% of doctors).

2. Data refer to all doctors licensed to practice (resulting in a large over-estimation of the number of practising doctors in Portugal, of around 30%).

Source: OECD Health Statistics 2015.

StatLink http://dx.doi.org/10.1787/888933325971

Similarly, the number of nurses has also increased in nearly all OECD countries, both in absolute number and on a per capita basis. This increase has occurred both in countries that had relatively low numbers in 2000 (such as Korea and Portugal) and in other countries that already had relatively high numbers (such as Switzerland, Norway and Denmark), although the growth rate has slowed down in some countries in the post-economic crisis period (such as Estonia, Ireland and Spain).

Figure 2. Rising numbers of nurses in OECD countries, 2000 and 2013 (or nearest year)

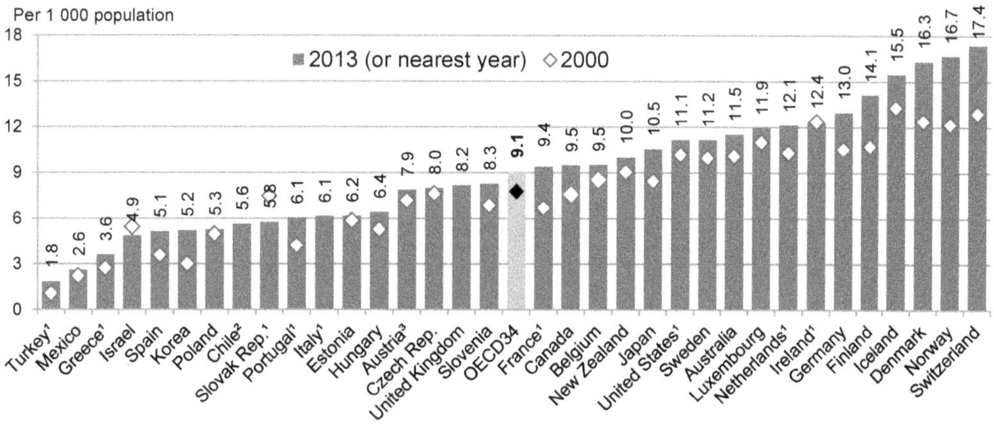

Information on data for Israel: http://dx.doi.org/10.1787/888932315602.

1. Data include not only nurses providing direct care to patients, but also those working in the health sector as managers, educators, researchers, etc.

2. Data in Chile refer to all nurses who are licensed to practice (less than one-third are professional nurses with a university degree).

3. Austria reports only nurses employed in hospital.

Source: OECD Health Statistics 2015.

StatLink http://dx.doi.org/10.1787/888933325986

The "skill mix" (or to be more precise, the occupational mix), as measured by the number of nurses per doctor, differs widely across OECD countries, reflecting different ways of organising health care delivery and the distribution of tasks among different health care providers. In half of the countries, there were between 2 to 4 nurses per doctor in 2013; yet, this ratio varied from less than one nurse per doctor in Greece to 4.5 nurses per doctor (or over) in Finland, Japan, Ireland and Denmark. Some countries (e.g., Finland, Ireland and the United States) clearly rely more on nurses to do some tasks that are still the prerogative of doctors or other health care providers in others.

Figure 3. Ratio of nurses per physician, OECD countries, 2013 (or nearest year)

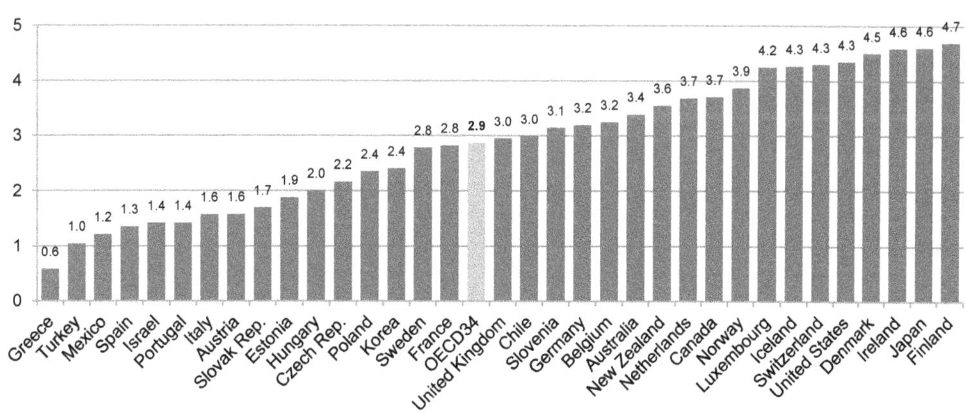

Information on data for Israel: http://dx.doi.org/10.1787/888932315602.

Source: OECD Health Statistics 2015.

StatLink http://dx.doi.org/10.1787/888933325992

2. Most OECD countries have increased their education and training efforts to address replacement needs and projected rising demand

One of the main policy levers that OECD countries can use to adjust the supply of health workers is to change their *numerus clausus* policies (the annual quotas) regarding the number of students admitted to medical, nursing and other health-related education programmes.

Most OECD countries have increased considerably student intakes in medical and nursing education programmes over the past decade, in response to concerns about current or future shortages and in some cases to become less reliant on the immigration of foreign-trained doctors and nurses. In Finland, France, Netherlands and United Kingdom, most of the increase in medical student intakes occurred in the early 2000s with the number stabilising afterwards, whereas in Australia, Canada, New Zealand, Portugal and Sweden, the increase continued steadily throughout the period.

Student admissions in nursing education have also expanded substantially in most OECD countries since 2000. In Australia, Ireland and the United States, admissions growth has been fairly rapid and steady throughout the period, also reflecting previous concerns about projected shortages. In the United States, student admissions in registered nurses (RN) education programmes doubled between 2001 and 2013 (rising from about 100 000 to 200 000 per year). This expansion in admissions in RN education programmes has increased so much that there are now concerns of an over-supply of new graduates. The most recent projections from the US Department of Health and Human Services in 2014 estimated that if student admission rates remain at their 2013 level, there might be an over-supply of more than 300 000 RNs by 2025.

The number of students admitted in medical education programmes in the United States has also increased, but at a slower rate than in nursing. Between 2001 and 2013, student intakes in US medical schools grew by over 33%. However, the number of residency posts has not increased at the same pace, creating a bottleneck.

Figure 4. The number of domestic medical and nursing graduates in the United States has increased more rapidly than the number of foreign-trained doctors and nurses

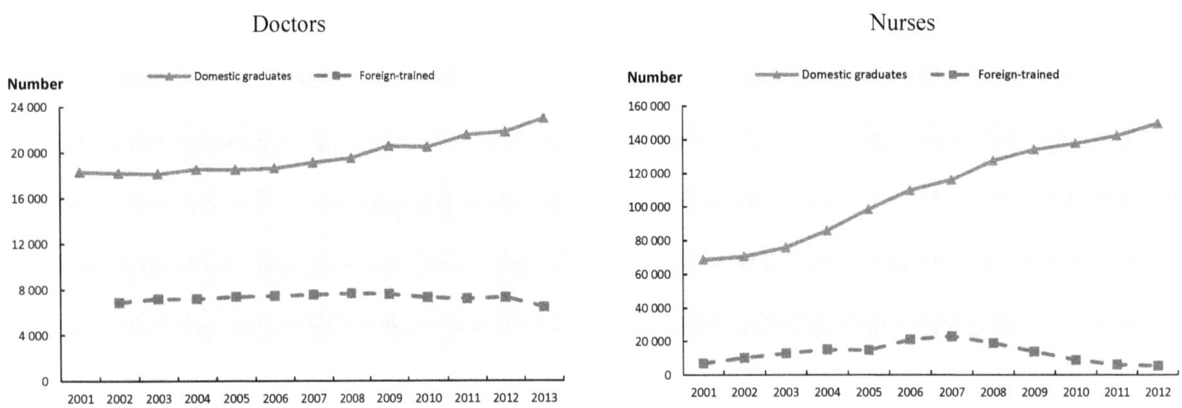

Source: The US Nursing Workforce: Trends in Supply and Education, Health Resources, Services Administration (HRSA), 2013; American Medical Associations, National Centre for Health Statistics.

StatLink http://dx.doi.org/10.1787/888933326324

In the United Kingdom, the rapid expansion of medical student intakes starting in the early 2000s was accompanied by a sharp reduction in the annual inflow of foreign-trained doctors from the peak reached in 2003 when health spending and the recruitment of doctors and other categories of health workers were growing very rapidly. The number of new graduates from nursing schools in the United Kingdom has also gone up over the past decade. This was accompanied by a sharp reduction in the inflow of foreign-trained nurses between 2004 and 2009. However, since then, the number of foreign-trained nurses has gone back up, driven mainly by the migration of nurses trained in other EU countries (e.g., Spain and Portugal) to meet unexpected demands for nurses. There are also large outflows of nurses trained in the United Kingdom towards Australia, Canada, New Zealand and the United States.

Figure 5. The number of domestic medical and nursing graduates in the United Kingdom has increased more rapidly than the number of foreign-trained doctors and nurses, United Kingdom

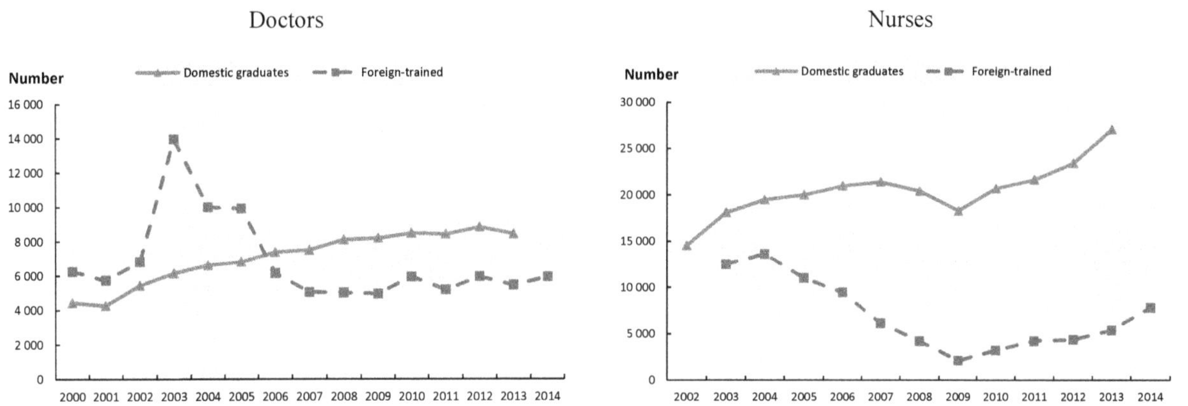

Note: Between 2005 and 2008, data on staff trained abroad correspond to the administrative period ending 31 March of the year indicated. Break in 2008 for the graduate series. Data from 2008 onwards are estimated.

Source: UK Graduate Output 1991/92 to 2012/13, Health and Social Care Information Centre. Nursing and Midwifery Council.

StatLink http://dx.doi.org/10.1787/888933326334

3. Some OECD countries have also started to train more general practitioners

There is growing consensus across OECD countries about the need to transform health systems that were initially created to deal mainly with acute care in hospital to better respond to the growing burden of chronic diseases by a team of providers outside the hospital. But although the overall number of doctors has gone up, the share of general practitioners (GPs) has continued to drop. On average across OECD countries, only one-third of doctors are generalists.

Figure 6. The share of generalists among all doctors has come down over the past 20 years

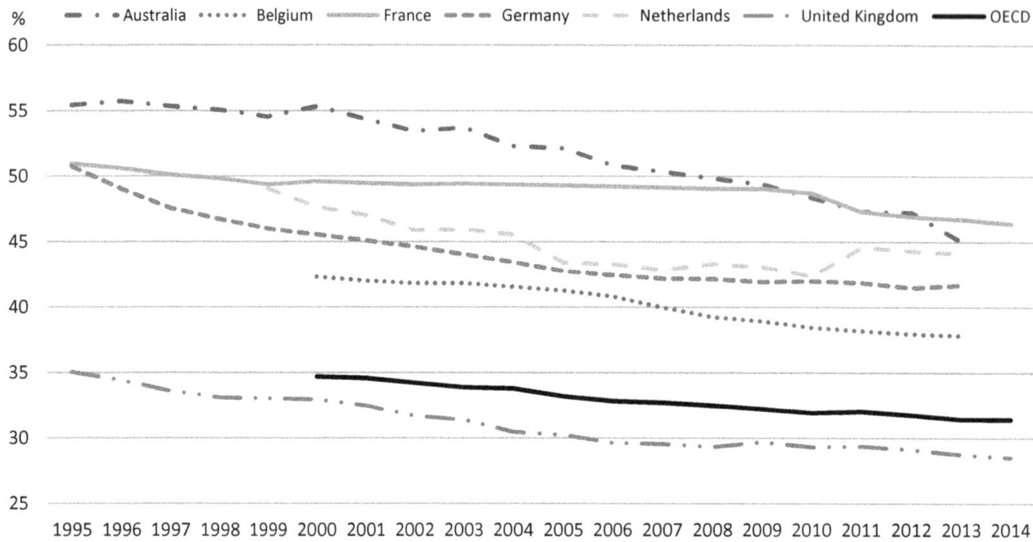

Note: Generalists include general practitioners ('family doctors') and other generalists (non-specialists).
Source: OECD Health Statistics 2015.

StatLink http://dx.doi.org/10.1787/888933326070

Several countries (e.g., Canada, France and the United Kingdom) have begun to take steps over the past decade to reverse this trend by increasing more rapidly the number of post-graduate training places in general medicine, although it has not always been easy to fill all the newly available places. A coherent and comprehensive strategy is needed to attract and retain more doctors to general medicine, including offering them clinical training places outside hospital, improving the relative remuneration of general practice, and reducing the workload and isolation still often associated with general practice by promoting group practices.

Some countries, for example the United States, Canada and the Netherlands, have increased student intakes in advanced education programmes for nurses, such as nurse practitioners (NPs) programmes, to increase the supply of "mid-level" providers. Many evaluations have shown that advanced practice nurses with proper training can improve access to primary care services and deliver the same quality of care as GPs for patients with minor illnesses, those with chronic conditions requiring routine follow-up, and others. Training and effectively using a greater number of advanced practice nurses may free up the time for doctors to deal with patients truly requiring medical diagnoses or treatments.

Too often however, there appears to be a lack of proper coordination in health workforce planning, and education and training policies, to assess in a more comprehensive way the future requirements of different categories of health workers. Health workforce planning and *numerus clausus* policies are still too often based on silo approaches, looking at each occupation in isolation.

4. Re-designing initial education and training programmes and strengthening continuous professional development to ensure that health workers have the right skills

Health professionals need a wide range of skills to perform their work efficiently, and these skills requirements are changing at a fast pace because of technological progress and new ways of delivering services. As in other sectors of the economy, there is not always a perfect match between the skills that health professionals have and the skills required in their jobs. Such skills mismatch raises concerns of a possible waste in human capital (when people are over-skilled for the work they do) or the quality and safety of health services (when they are lacking certain skills).

Based on the 2011-12 Programme for International Assessment of Adult Competencies (PIAAC) survey, about 50% of doctors reported being under-skilled for some of the tasks that they have to do, a much higher share than workers in other occupations. At the same time, the vast majority of doctors and nurses also reported being over-skilled for some of the work that they have to do.

Figure 7. Reported under-skilling by physicians, nurses and other occupations, PIAAC Survey, 2011-12

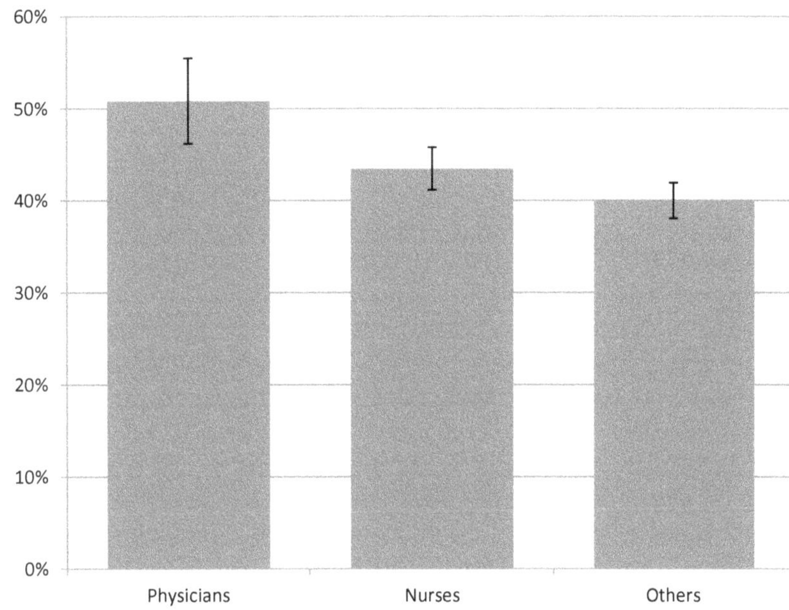

Note: Others = workers in other technical and professional occupations (ISCO 2 and 3). The figure depicts percentage responses with the associated 95% confidence interval.

Source: PIAAC, OECD analysis.

StatLink http://dx.doi.org/10.1787/888933326509

A crucial issue to make sure that future generations of doctors and nurses will have the right skills to be "fit for practice" is the design of initial medical and nursing education programmes, since it is during these formative years that they will acquire a large part of the skills that they will use throughout their professional lives. Training of health professionals for the 21st century calls for more attention to team-based training of different health professionals and problem-based learning to overcome current gaps between the skills acquired in schools and the requirements in the workplaces.

Figure 8. Reported over-skilling by physicians, nurses and other occupations, PIAAC Survey, 2011-12

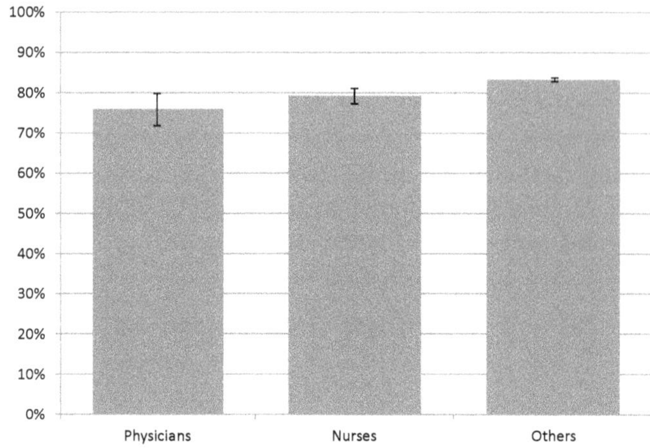

Note: Others = workers in other technical and professional occupations (ISCO 2 and 3). The figure depicts percentage responses with the associated 95% confidence interval.

Source: PIAAC, OECD analysis.

StatLink http://dx.doi.org/10.1787/888933326492

Continuous professional development (CPD) is another important policy lever to ensure that the skills of practising doctors and nurses are kept up-to-date in a context of changing technologies and job requirements. In at least a dozen of OECD countries, participation in CPD activities for doctors is combined with re-licensing or re-registration requirements, as part of important health workforce management processes to ensure quality and patient safety. There is growing recognition that awarding a license to practise at the end of initial medical or nursing education is not sufficient to ensure high quality of care throughout the working life, considering the rapidly changing nature of health care delivery. Policies and regulations concerning CPD vary greatly across OECD countries. There are variations notably regarding whether participation in CPD activities is mandatory or not, whether there are requirements for health professionals to renew their licenses or registrations, and where that is the case, whether a certain amount of CPD is a mandatory part of the re-licensing or re-registration process. In the United Kingdom, CPD is linked to re-licensing or re-registration protocols, although CPD provisions for doctors do not follow a uniform nation-wide system.

Regardless of whether mandatory or voluntary systems are in place, some key common barriers to greater participation in CPD activities for doctors, nurses and other health professionals are lack of time and related cost. There is a need for more systematic and organisational support to allow professionals to take time off for CPD and to ensure that the costs are not prohibitive.

Policies also need to address over-skilling, which is reported by more than 70% of doctors and nurses who participated in the 2011-12 PIAAC survey. These policies involve reviewing the scope of practice of different health care providers, with a view to promote a fuller use of their skills and to delegate down some tasks that might be performed by "mid-level" providers or lower-skilled workers (such as health care assistants). Results from the 2011-12 PIAAC survey indicate that nurses with an advanced university degree are much more likely to report being over-skilled for the job they do compared to those with a bachelor's or lower degree.

At least one-third of OECD countries reported in 2012-13 that they had introduced or expanded the roles of non-physician providers in the previous five years to improve access to care, particularly in primary care. These include promoting more advanced roles for nurses, as well as pharmacists and other providers. Past experience in the United States, Canada and Nordic countries shows that advanced practice nurses can play a particularly useful role to address the needs of population in areas underserved by doctors. However, the introduction or expansion of more advanced roles for nurses often needs to overcome the initial opposition from the medical profession.

5. Using technology and innovative health service delivery models to provide proper access to care for people living in rural and remote regions

A persisting major policy issue in many OECD countries is the uneven distribution of doctors across different geographic regions, which may limit access to primary care and hospital care for populations living in rural and remote regions (who often have greater health needs because they are older and sicker). This issue is particularly important in geographically-large countries, like Australia, Canada, the United States and the Nordic countries.

In all countries, the number of physicians per capita is greater in urban regions (and particularly in national capital regions) than in rural areas, reflecting the preference of physicians to practise in urban settings and the greater concentration of specialist services.

A wide range of policies have been tried in different OECD countries to address this issue, with uneven success:

- *Policies targeting the selection of medical students or the location of medical schools:* Policies focussing on student selection are based on evidence that students coming from rural backgrounds have a greater likelihood to practice in rural areas once they have completed their training than those coming from urban areas. Australia and Japan have fixed some minimum quota of medical places reserved for students with a rural background, sometimes accompanied by financial support provided to these students or any other students in exchange for a return-of-service obligation to practice for a number of years in underserved areas once they have completed their training. Norway, Japan and Canada have established some medical schools in rural or remote regions, with the expectation that more students graduating from these schools would remain in these regions afterwards. There is evidence from these countries that a high proportion of students stay in these rural/remote regions, even though some additional financial incentives are also sometime provided.
- *Providing financial incentives for doctors to practice in underserved areas or implementing regulations to restrict the choice of practice location:* Another common approach is to provide various types of financial incentives to attract doctors to practice in underserved areas and to retain them, for example through one-off payments to facilitate their installation and/or recurrent supplementary payments or bonuses. In Germany, most states (*Länder*) offer financial incentives for GPs who are opening their practice for the first time, with GPs eligible to a higher payment if they choose to locate in underserved areas. This is combined with regulations which restrict the freedom of doctors to set up a new practice in areas that are deemed to be adequately supplied. Australia steers international medical graduates and foreign-trained physicians into underserved areas, using regulations to impose practice in designated areas for a number of years.

Figure 9. The number of doctors varies widely across regions (2013 or nearest year)

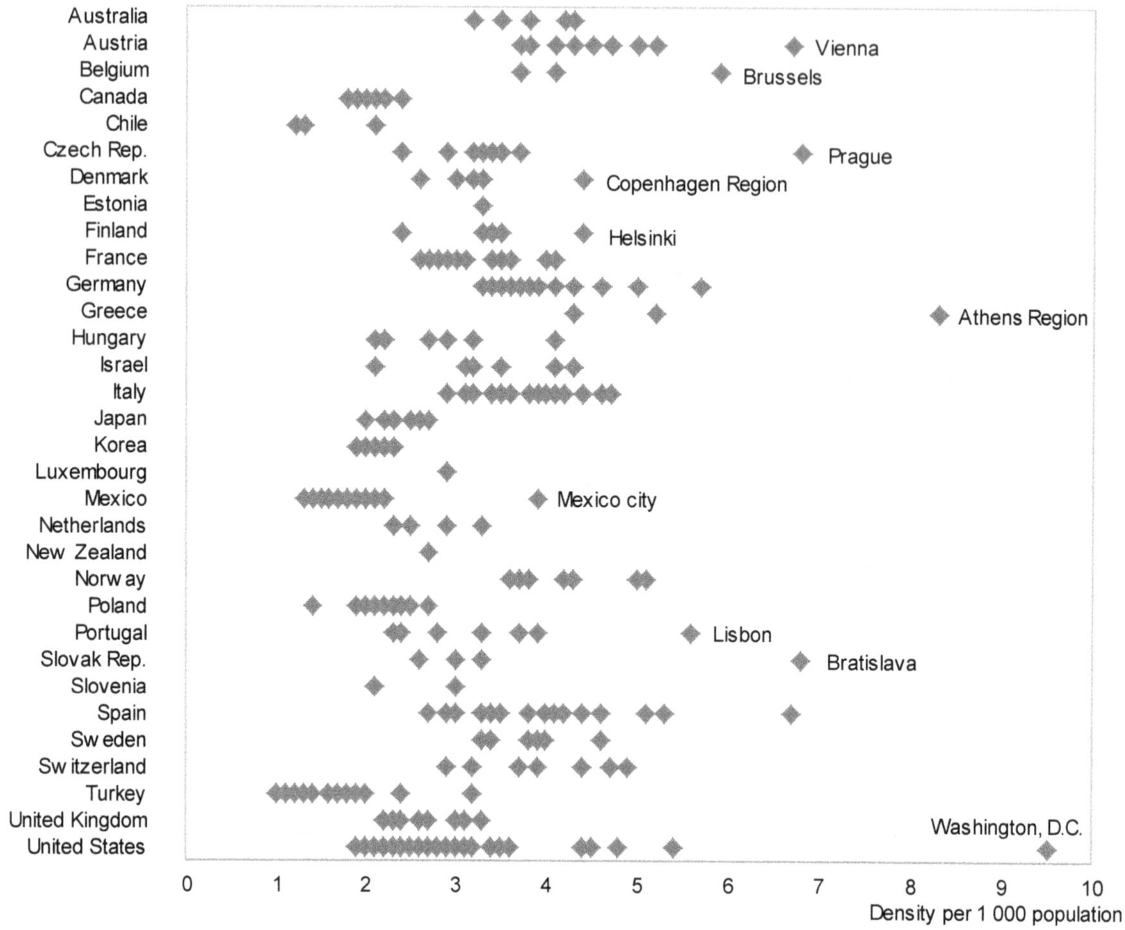

Note: Each observation (point) represents a territorial level 2 region (for example, *region* in France, *Länder* in Germany or *State* in the United States) in each country. The data for Chile relate to 2009 and do not reflect the increase in the number of physicians since then.

Information on data for Israel: http://dx.doi.org/10.1787/888932315602.

Source: OECD (2015), *Health at a Glance 2015: OECD Indicators,* OECD Publishing, Paris, http://dx.doi.org/10.1787/health_glance-2015-en.

StatLink http://dx.doi.org/10.1787/888933326402

- *Promoting innovations in health service delivery and telemedicine:* Many countries have also promoted various types of innovations in health service delivery to achieve the goal of providing adequate access to services with fewer doctors on site. These innovations include encouraging a transfer of competences from doctors to nurses and other local health professionals, and the development of telemedicine to connect patients and doctors through remote distance when needed. Telemedicine can also be used to connect local nurses and other paramedical staff with doctors to seek advice and support on diagnoses and prescriptions as needed. There are growing numbers of initiatives underway across OECD countries to exploit the use of telemedicine to improve access to health services, notably in large countries such as Canada, Australia and Finland, but also in smaller size countries such as Portugal.

These policy levers are not mutually exclusive and may have a greater impact if they are used in combination. The French Ministry of Health and Social Affairs has launched in 2012 a fairly comprehensive "Health Territory Pact" to promote the recruitment and retention of doctors in underserved areas and innovative ways of delivering services in these locations which combines many of the above-mentioned policies. This Pact contains a series of measures to encourage the establishment of young doctors in underserved regions, including not only financial incentives but also improvements in their working conditions notably through the creation of new multi-disciplinary medical homes allowing physicians and other health professionals to work in the same location. It also includes the promotion of telemedicine and the transfer of competences from doctors to other local health care providers.

6. Reducing the reliance on foreign-trained health workers

The international migration of skilled workers is not unique to the health sector, but it continues to raise serious concerns when it is exacerbating shortages of skilled health workers in those countries (notably low-income countries) that are already suffering from even more acute shortages. When they adopted the Global Code of Practice on the International Recruitment of Health Personnel in 2010, all WHO members committed to improving their health workforce planning and to respond to their future needs without relying unduly on the training efforts of other countries. The goal is not necessarily to achieve self-sufficiency, but to avoid relying systematically on other countries to fill domestic needs by training a sufficient number domestically.

The marked increase in domestic education and training efforts in many OECD countries over the past decade has already reduced considerably the inflows of foreign-trained doctors and nurses moving to these countries. This is notably the case in the United States – the biggest importer of foreign-trained doctors and nurses – where the inflows of foreign-trained nurses in particular is now much lower compared to what it was ten years ago (Figure 4). In the United Kingdom (the second biggest importer), the number of new domestic medical graduates now exceeds the number of foreign-trained doctors as the main source of new inflows in the health system. The composition of foreign-trained doctors has also changed considerably over the past decade, with fewer doctors coming from Africa and Asia, and a growing number of doctors coming from other EU countries.

Within the EU, there have been large emigrations of doctors and nurses from some of the new EU member countries in Central and Eastern Europe to Western Europe following their accession, as barriers to mobility were reduced notably through the mutual recognition of professional qualifications. In some cases, this emigration has seriously affected the supply of health workers, particularly in rural areas which were already lacking skilled health workers. To address this expatriation issue, several Central and Eastern European countries have introduced measures to increase the retention of doctors and nurses by increasing salaries and improving working conditions, despite tight budget constraints.

Consistent with the broad principles of the WHO Global Code of Practice, some OECD countries have reached since 2010 some bilateral or multilateral agreements with other countries to achieve mutually beneficial cooperation in international training and recruitment of health personnel. Up to now, these bilateral or multilateral agreements have involved only a fairly limited number of doctors and nurses, but these cooperation agreements might expand in the future particularly if they are steered towards positions that are hard to fill in receiving countries.

7. Conclusions

As with all areas of human endeavour, the provision of health care is continually changing, driven by innovation, technology, the changing health needs of populations, and economic constraints. While this has always been the case, the rate of change is accelerating. These changes present tremendous opportunities to deliver better and more efficient health services to more people. At the same time, they are also a challenge for health systems and the traditional functions and responsibilities of health professionals. Policy makers, professional groups, educational institutions and citizens need to work together to overcome these challenges and ensure health systems continue to meet changing needs and rising expectations.

Health workforce planning and policies in many OECD countries have been confronted with the short-term goal of ensuring that there will be a sufficient number of the conventional health care providers that have traditionally played a central role in health systems (notably doctors and nurses), with the longer-term objective of promoting necessary transformations in health service delivery models to better respond to changing population health needs and better exploit new technologies and the skills of various providers. In responding to pressures to achieve the short-term goal, policy-makers need to make sure that the decisions will not make it more difficult to achieve this longer-term objective.

Looking ahead, health workforce policies should be designed to achieve the goal of having the right number and mix of health care providers, with the right skills, providing services in the right places, to better respond to changing population health needs and ensure good value for the growing amount of money spent on health.

The right jobs

- Countries need to *train a sufficient number and proper mix of health workers* to meet future needs. They should pursue this goal without "free-riding" on the training efforts of other countries, particularly those suffering from acute shortages.
- Countries need to optimise the scope of practice of different health care providers, with a view to make the best use of their *qualifications and skills*. They need to remove any unnecessary barriers to the full scope of practice and promote innovative and collaborative health service delivery models to meet changing population health needs.

The right skills

- Countries need to *ensure that health workers acquire and maintain the right skills and competences* to deliver high-quality health services in more team-based and patient-centred approaches. In a context of rapidly changing technologies and evolving health service delivery models, there is a need to adapt education and training programmes, encourage continuous professional development and the regular re-certification of health professionals to ensure that their skills are kept up-to-date.

The right places

- Countries need to ensure that all the population has adequate access to health care regardless of where they live, by promoting a more even geographic distribution of health workers through financial incentives and/or regulations, enabling broader scopes of practice for non-physician providers with the required training and skills, and making greater use of innovative health service delivery models, notably telemedicine.

Chapter 1
Analytical framework of health labour markets

By Gaétan Lafortune (OECD Health Division)

This first chapter takes a broad look at how health labour markets function. It presents a general framework for analysing the range of factors affecting both the supply of, and demand for, health workers. The discussion starts by presenting a basic supply framework, and then adds other components on both the supply and demand side. In all OECD countries, the functioning of the labour market for doctors, nurses and other health professionals is characterised by strong government interventions, affecting both the supply and the demand sides. The main rationale put forward for these government interventions is also discussed.

1.1. Introduction

Health workers play a central role in delivering a wide range of health services to the population. For decades now, most of the policy and public discourse on health workforce issues has centred around the issue of shortages of health workers, notably of doctors and nurses as the main health care providers in most OECD countries. In many countries, particularly those that are geographically large, there have also been persisting concerns about the uneven geographic distribution of doctors and other health workers, particularly in rural and remote regions, and a wide range of measures have been taken to promote adequate access to care to people wherever they live. There have also been on-going concerns about a "brain drain" of skilled health workers moving from lower-income to higher-income countries, thereby often exacerbating the shortages of health workers in those countries that need them the most. More recently, there has been growing interest in many OECD countries to review the scope of practice of non-physician providers and to develop new professional roles, with a view to improve access to care and promote a more efficient use of human resources.

In all OECD countries, the functioning of the labour market for doctors, nurses and other health workers is characterised by strong government interventions, affecting both the supply and the demand sides. On the supply side, the range of government interventions typically include: the subsidisation of medical, nursing and other health-related education programmes, often combined with quotas on the number of students admitted each year (through so-called *numerus clausus* policies); regulations around the (re-)licensing and (re-)registration of doctors, nurses and other health professionals allowing them to practice, often justified on the grounds of patient safety; a range of policies that might be used to influence the geographic distribution of health workers (including both financial incentives and regulations around the choice of practice location – so-called "carrots" and "sticks"); and policies affecting the immigration of foreign health workers (including the recognition of their qualifications and skills). Government interventions also play a very important role regarding the demand for doctors, nurses and other health workers, given that most health spending in nearly all OECD countries is publicly funded.[1] Government policies related to public coverage of different health services and goods, the level and growth rate in public spending on health and the direct employment of health workers in NHS-type systems in some countries can all have important effects on the demand for different categories of health workers.

This first chapter of the publication outlines some general considerations in analysing the functioning of health labour markets and policy impacts. It presents a general framework for the analyses of the range of factors that affect both the supply and demand for health workers. The discussion starts by presenting a basic supply framework, and then adds other components on both the supply and demand side. The main rationale put forward for government interventions on both the supply and demand side is also discussed.

1.2. The supply of health workers

Figure 1.1 starts by presenting a basic framework to look at some of the main factors affecting the supply of health workers. It is based on a classic stock/flow model, where changes over time in the stock (or supply) of health workers is affected by inflows (which depend mainly on the entry of new graduates in the workforce and the immigration of foreign-trained workers) and outflows (including people leaving the workforce because of retirement or for other reasons, and the emigration of some workers to other countries).

The supply of health workers is not only determined by the number of people working in the system, but also by their working hours (or activity rates). The number of hours that health professionals work is influenced by many factors, including the demand for their services (e.g., working overtime when the demand is strong), their pay rates (with the assumption under the conventional labour market theory that higher hourly pay rates will increase working hours, although the reality may be more complex) and other aspects of working conditions (which may positively or negatively affect working hours).

Figure 1.1. Basic framework for the supply of health workers: Stock/flow model

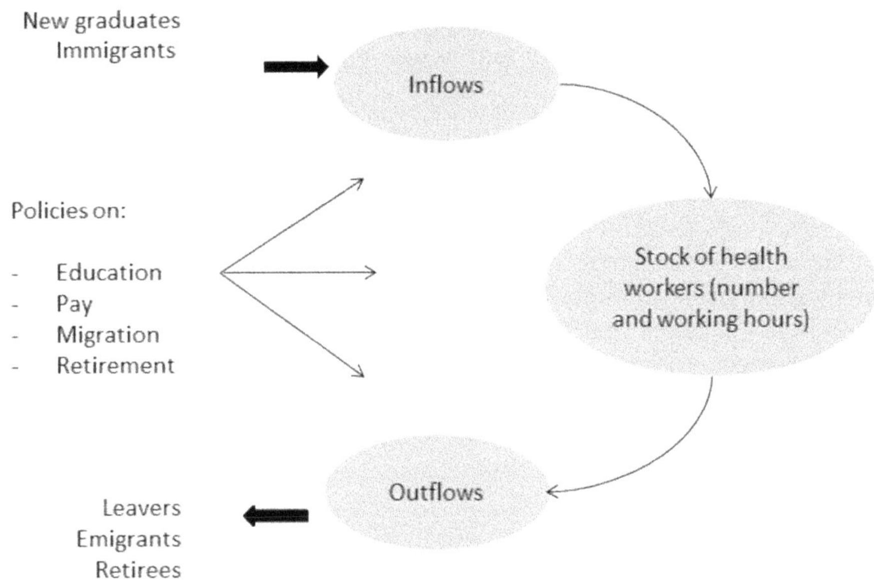

A range of policies may affect the supply of health workers, including the inflows, activity rates and retention rates (outflows). For example, all OECD countries subsidise medical education and in nearly all countries this is also accompanied by the setting of quantitative limits to the number of students admitted each year, so-called *numerus clausus* policies. The rationale for limiting the number of students in medical education programmes through some *numerus clausus* policies includes: to limit entry in medical schools to the most able applicants, to restrain direct public expenditure for medical education, and to control the total number of doctors for cost-containment reasons (as greater supply may induce greater demand). As noted in Chapter 3, the *numerus clausus* is a very powerful policy lever that governments can use to adjust either upwards or downwards the supply of doctors, nurses and other health professionals, although there is a time lag of several years between the time that a decision is made to increase (or decrease) student intakes and the impact on entry into the health workforce.

Beyond adjusting their education policy, governments may also open up or tighten their immigration policy to recruit more or fewer health professionals from other countries. The recruitment of foreign-trained doctors and nurses may be able to respond more quickly to any current shortages than any changes in education policy.

All OECD countries regulate entry in medical and other health professions through some form of licensing and registration, with this responsibility often delegated to medical councils or other professional organisations. The main rationale for requiring such licensing and registration (and in some cases also re-registration during professional lives) is to ensure that health care providers meet certain minimum standards in terms of theoretical and practical skills and competences to ensure a certain level of quality of care and patient safety. However, one of the possible downsides to such licensing and registration procedures is that these create barriers to entry in these professions, possibly allowing those who are in the professions to benefit from rents (i.e., higher remunerations than would have otherwise been the case in a free labour market without any barrier to entry).

Governments can also influence the activity rates and retention rates of health workers through policies related to working time (e.g., a reduction in the maximum number of working hours per week will reduce the supply of services), pay rates and retirement policies. Adjustments to pay rates can have both short-term and longer-term effects on the number of people working in health systems and on their working hours. For example, pay raises for nurses may increase their retention rates and their working hours in the short term, and increase the attractiveness of the profession in the longer term. In a context of increasing international migration, any meaningful remuneration gap between the health professionals working in one country compared to other countries may also provide some financial incentives for people to move to countries where they may be able to receive a higher pay, particularly if barriers to mobility between countries are low or almost inexistent. Differences in payment methods (for example, salary, capitation payments, or fee-for-services payments for doctors) can also be expected to have an impact on working hours and activity rates.

1.3. The demand for health workers

Many factors affect the demand for health services. Figure 1.2 adds to the previous framework some of the main drivers of demand for health workers, applied here to physicians (but the same factors would also influence the demand for nurses and other health care providers). These factors include: overall economic development and economic growth and the share of GDP allocated to health spending (which influences the ability to pay health workers from public or private sources), demographic factors (including population size and structure), and morbidity (the incidence/prevalence of various diseases and injuries).

The organisation of health service delivery can also influence the demand for different categories of health workers by affecting the skill mix and occupation mix. Figure 1.2 shows that there are many possible forms of interactions and substitutions among different categories of health workers in delivering health services. The demand for physician services (GPs or specialists) is partly driven by the availability of other human resources (e.g., nurses), which may either complement or substitute for the services delivered by physicians. Government policies can affect the composition of the health workforce in a number of ways, notably through public funding for education and training programmes for different categories of doctors, nurses and other health professionals, and through implementing regulatory changes in their scope of practice.

Figure 1.2. Framework for the supply and demand for health workers (applied to physicians)

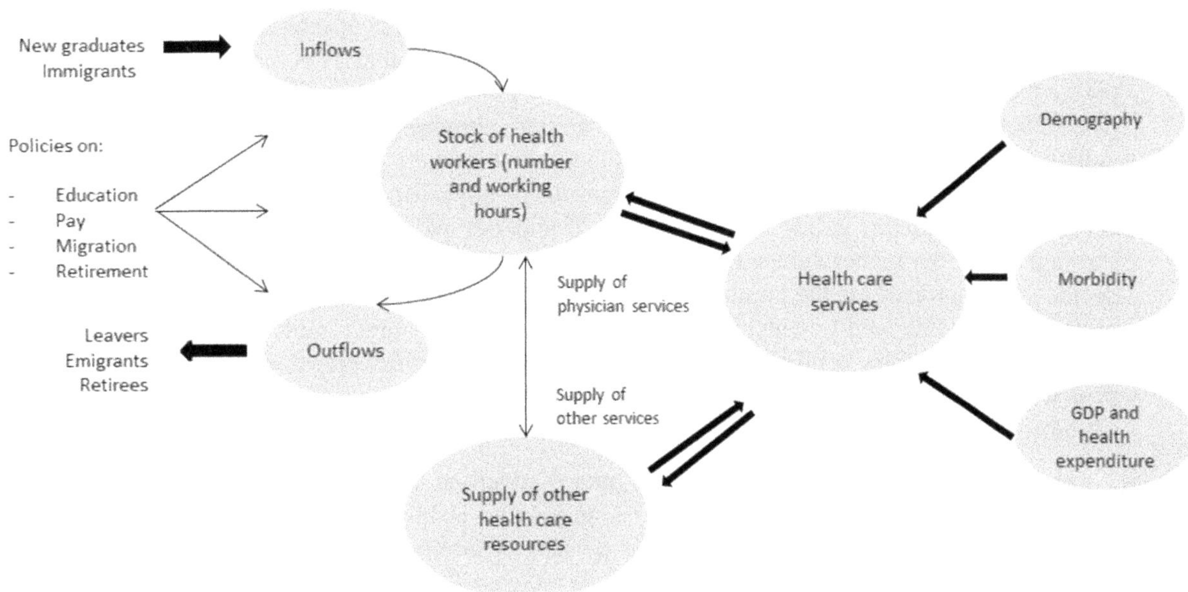

1.4. The search for equilibrium in health labour markets

Most of the discussions on health workforce issues in OECD countries over the past decades have focussed on the issue of shortages, suggesting that there is some form of "permanent disequilibrium" on these labour markets. But how might it be that the labour market for doctors, nurses and other health care providers never reach equilibrium (i.e., a balance between demand and supply)?

According to standard economic theory, the labour market for different categories of health workers should reach equilibrium mainly through wage adjustments. The assumption is that, when wages go up, so does supply (either in terms of the number of health workers and/or their working hours) while the demand decreases, and vice-versa. This wage adjustment is shown theoretically in Figure 1.3. The example shown here assumes that there is an initial equilibrium between the demand and supply of doctors (depicted as the point Q_a in terms of full-time equivalent doctors and P_a in terms of their average wage). This point in equilibrium is disrupted by an upward shift in demand triggered, for instance, by a rise in GDP and health expenditure, which shifts the demand from D_a to D_b. If the supply of doctors is not perfectly elastic (which is likely to be the case given the time that it takes to train new doctors), the prices for their services (wages or fees) should in theory increase. If this occurs, in the short term, the supply response to the higher demand might come mainly from current workers choosing to work more hours in return for higher (hourly) wages (for instance, more doctors, nurses and other health professionals working overtime). However, in the medium to longer-term, any increase in pay rates (wages or fees) might be expected to attract more people in the profession (e.g., more foreign-trained doctors or more new domestic graduates), moving the supply curve from S_a to S_b. The new equilibrium in this simplified model would be reached at point Q_b and P_b, the end result being that there is a greater number of doctors working in the system and earning higher wages to respond to the greater demand.

In reality, both the pay rates and quantities of services provided in health labour markets are not perfectly elastic, not only because of the time that it takes to train new doctors in response to any changes in demand, but also because of government interventions in these markets. One characteristic of health labour markets in many countries is the "monopsony" power that may be exercised by the dominant public purchaser on the price paid for doctor (and other health worker) services. For illustration purposes, let's assume that public authorities have set the wages or fees for doctors for many years at an intermediate wage, P_c. In this scenario, there would be a surplus of physicians under the initial demand curve D_a (some doctors would be unemployed or under-employed), while there would be a shortage under the higher demand curve D_b. If such a shortage emerges, governments may decide to further increase the number of doctors (by further increasing the *numerus clausus* in medical studies or by relaxing immigration policies to attract more foreign-trained doctors) to reach a new equilibrium at the point $Q_f - P_c$. Otherwise, they could also increase their wages or fees in the hope that this would increase their working hours to reach a new equilibrium at the point $Q_b - P_b$.[2]

How elastic is the supply of working time of doctors, nurses and other health care providers to changes in their pay rates? The supply curve shown in Figure 1.3 assumes a continuously upward slope – as the wages or fees of doctors (or any other health care providers) increase, it is assumed that they will increase their work effort. However, it is also possible that after a certain point, the supply curve may be backward-bending, if the "substitution" effect (a preference for more leisure) exceeds the "income" effect. Following a review of a number of studies in different countries, Nicholson and Propper (2012) concluded that changes in wages (or fees) do not appear to have any strong effect on physicians or nurses work effort (i.e., the income effect is small). The implication is that the response to any increase in demand for their services will need to come mainly by increasing the number of health workers in the system.

Figure 1.3. Derived demand for and supply of physicians

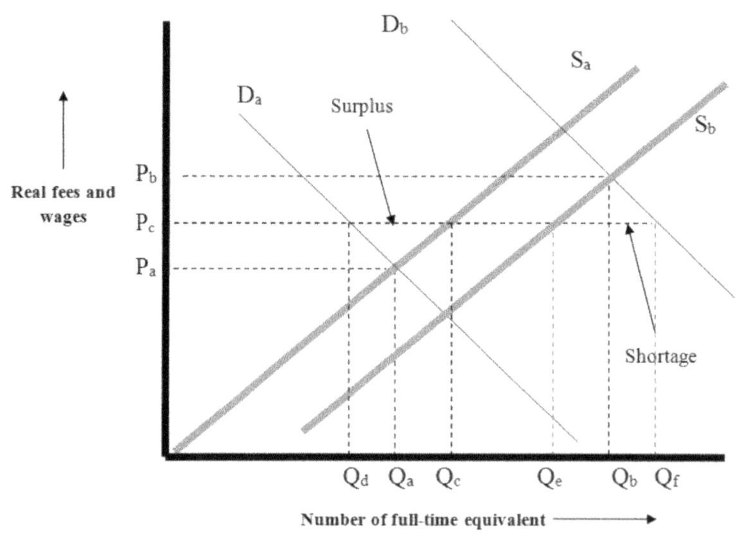

1.5. Conclusions

The brief theoretical discussion and frameworks presented in this first chapter provide a starting point to analyse recent trends in the demand for and the supply of different categories of health workers, and the impact of government policies on those. Chapter 2 discusses some of these broad trends and policy priorities in OECD countries following the economic crisis in 2008, which led to a marked slowdown or reduction in health spending in many countries and a re-orientation of policy priorities. Chapter 3 focusses specifically on recent policy changes regarding education and training programmes for doctors and nurses – the main policy lever that governments have to influence the future supply of health workers. Chapter 4 reviews recent trends in the other main source of inflows in medical and nursing professions – the migration of foreign-trained doctors and nurses in OECD countries, including also a review of some of the policies that some countries have adopted to reduce the outflow (emigration) of skilled workers. The demand and supply of different categories of health workers may vary widely not only across countries, but also across different geographic areas in each country. Chapter 5 describes and assesses the range of policies that many OECD countries have adopted to promote a better geographic distribution of doctors and health services within their country, particularly in rural and remote areas. Chapter 6 addresses issues regarding skills use and the extent of skills mismatch in the health sector, and possible policy options to address issues of over-skilling or under-skilling to promote greater efficiency and quality in health service delivery.

Notes

1. In 2013, nearly three-quarters of health spending was publicly-funded on average across OECD countries (OECD, 2015).

2. Another option (not shown in Figure 1.3) may also be to substitute some doctors by extending the role of other health care providers in areas where there are shortages of doctors.

References

Nicholson, S. and C. Propper (2012), *Handbook of Health Economics*, Vol. 2, 2, edited by M. Pauly, T. McGuire and P. Pito Barros, Elsevier, Amsterdam.

OECD (2015), *OECD Health Statistics 2015*, OECD Publishing, Paris, http://www.oecd.org/els/health-systems/health-data.htm.

Ono, T., G. Lafortune and M. Schoenstein (2013), "Health Workforce Planning in OECD Countries: A Review of 26 Health Workforce Projection Models from 18 Countries", *OECD Health Working Papers*, No. 62, OECD Publishing, Paris, http://dx.doi.org/10.1787/5k44t787zcwb-en.

Chapter 2
Trends in health labour markets and policy priorities to address workforce issues

By Gaétan Lafortune, Michael Schoenstein and Liliane Moreira
(OECD Health Division)[1]

Prior to the economic crisis, there were widespread concerns in most OECD countries about a looming crisis in the health workforce. Growing shortages of health workers were expected to result from the retirement of the "baby-boom" generation of doctors and nurses and from steady increases in the demand for their services from an ageing population. However, these concerns have since lessened considerably in many OECD countries as countries have adapted their education and training policies leading to a growing supply of new doctors and nurses, and retention rates have also increased. This chapter describes recent trends in health labour markets in OECD countries before, during and following the economic crisis in terms of employment levels and remuneration rates, and considers key policy priorities of OECD countries in health workforce development and management. It finds that the employment of doctors and nurses has continued to increase both in absolute number and on a per capita basis, although the demand in some countries did not grow as quickly as expected following reductions in health spending after the crisis. The main health workforce priorities in many OECD countries have evolved from general concerns about widespread shortages to more specific issues regarding the mix and geographic distribution of certain categories of workers.

2.1. Introduction

In most OECD countries, prior to the economic crisis there were widespread concerns about growing shortages of doctors and nurses arising from the retirement of the "baby-boom" generation of doctors and nurses, as well as a steady increase in the demand for their services linked to both growing income and population ageing. However, these concerns have lessened considerably. Contrary to the pre-crisis projections in many countries, the supply of doctors and nurses has not decreased in recent years, while the demand for doctors and nurses did not grow as quickly as expected.

In 2013, there were more employed doctors and nurses (in absolute number and on a per capita basis) in nearly all OECD countries than prior to the crisis. This increase in supply has been driven by three factors: 1) a rise in the number of students admitted and graduating from medical and nursing schools in most countries (which is discussed in more detail in Chapter 3); 2) a marked increase in the retention rates and the retirement age of many doctors and nurses, thereby reducing the exit rates; and 3) an increase in the number of foreign-trained doctors and nurses in some OECD countries (discussed in more detail in Chapter 4). At the same time, following the economic crisis, in many countries the demand for certain categories of health workers slowed down, at least temporarily, as health budgets were cut down in response to growing budgetary deficits.

The number of students admitted in medical and nursing education programmes has continued to increase in many OECD countries even after the economic crisis. This rise has been driven, at least partly, by continued concerns regarding the large wave of doctors and nurses who are approaching retirement age. The results from an expansion in student intakes are not felt immediately, as the length of the education and training periods, particularly for doctors, can take around ten years. Graduation rates over the coming years are therefore already known with a fairly high degree of certainty, with most OECD countries set for further increases in graduate numbers. At the same time, the likelihood of health professionals leaving their jobs has decreased in recent years, probably due to a combination of cyclical factors (related to the recession, which may only be temporary) and structural ones (which may have long lasting effects).

In this new context, the main policy priorities on health workforce have shifted from broad concerns about widespread shortages of doctors and nurses towards more specific issues. These new priorities include the imbalance in the medical workforce (notably the declining share of general practitioners), the under-supply of health workers in certain geographic regions, and opportunities and challenges to extend the roles for non-physician providers to improve access to care and efficiency in health service delivery. Many countries have taken steps recently to introduce or expand the roles of non-physician providers, such as nurse practitioners (NPs) or pharmacists, to maintain or increase access to health services in a cost-efficient way. Such changes in scope of practice can be expected to have an impact on future staffing requirements. Health workforce planning and management needs to better integrate recent developments affecting the supply and demand for health workers, and possible substitutions of tasks between different professional groups.

Section 2.2 of this chapter provides an overview of recent trends in employment levels and remuneration rates of health workers in OECD countries following the economic crisis, focussing on doctors and nurses. Section 2.3 describes the main policy priorities related to health workforce development and management as identified by health ministries in their response to the *2012 OECD Health System Characteristics Survey*.

2.2. Health workforce trends in OECD countries

This section starts by providing a brief overview of the impact of the 2008-09 economic crisis on GDP growth and overall unemployment rates in different OECD countries. Next, it compares the evolution of total employment with employment in the health and social sector during that same period in some countries. It then examines trends in employment levels of doctors and nurses before and after the economic crisis based on the results from the OECD/Eurostat/WHO-Europe Joint Questionnaire related to health employment and education. The trends in remuneration rates are based on a separate OECD data collection.

Macro-economic trends

On average across OECD countries, GDP fell by nearly 5% in real terms during the 2008-09 economic crisis. While the recession was widespread, its scale varied significantly across OECD countries. In 2008-09, real GDP declined from peak-to-trough by less than 1% in Poland and Australia, whereas it went down by more than 10% in Estonia, Iceland, Ireland and Finland. The economic recovery since then has also been very uneven. In the time period from its lowest point during the 2008-09 crisis to the first quarter in 2014, real GDP increased by more than 15% in Chile, Korea, Israel, Estonia, Mexico, Australia and Sweden, whereas growth remained negative during this time period in Greece (-21%), Portugal, Spain, Italy and Slovenia (Figure 2.1).

Figure 2.1. Reduction in GDP during the great recession in 2008-09 and change in GDP in following years (up to first quarter 2014), OECD countries

Percentage change in real GDP during the crisis (from GDP peak to GDP trough) and the early recovery (from GDP trough to 2014 Q1) in OECD countries

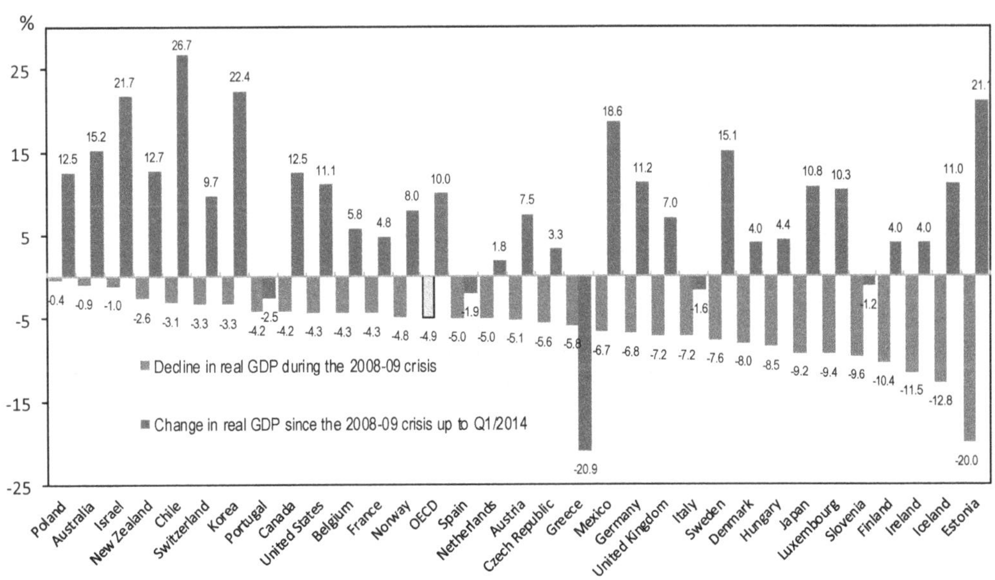

Note: When the change in real GDP during the recovery is higher (lower) than the decline in real GDP during the global financial crisis, then the real GDP level in 2014 Q1 is higher (lower) than its pre-crisis level.

Source: OECD calculations based on the OECD Economic Outlook Database.

StatLink http://dx.doi.org/10.1787/888933325947

The unemployment rate soared in many countries following the onset of the economic crisis in 2008. On average across OECD countries, the unemployment rate rose from 6% in 2008 to over 8% in 2009 and 2010, and remained at close to 8% in 2011, 2012 and 2013. As with GDP growth, the rise in unemployment rate varied greatly across OECD countries. In a majority of countries, the unemployment rate in 2013 was higher than in 2007 before the crisis (Figure 2.2). This was particularly the case in Southern European countries which by 2013 had not yet experienced any economic recovery. The overall unemployment rate in Greece and Spain reached more than 25% in 2013. The rate was also high in Portugal, the Slovak Republic and Ireland, although in the latter two countries the rate was coming down from its earlier peak (Figure 2.2).

Figure 2.2. Unemployment rate, OECD countries, 2007, 2010 and 2013

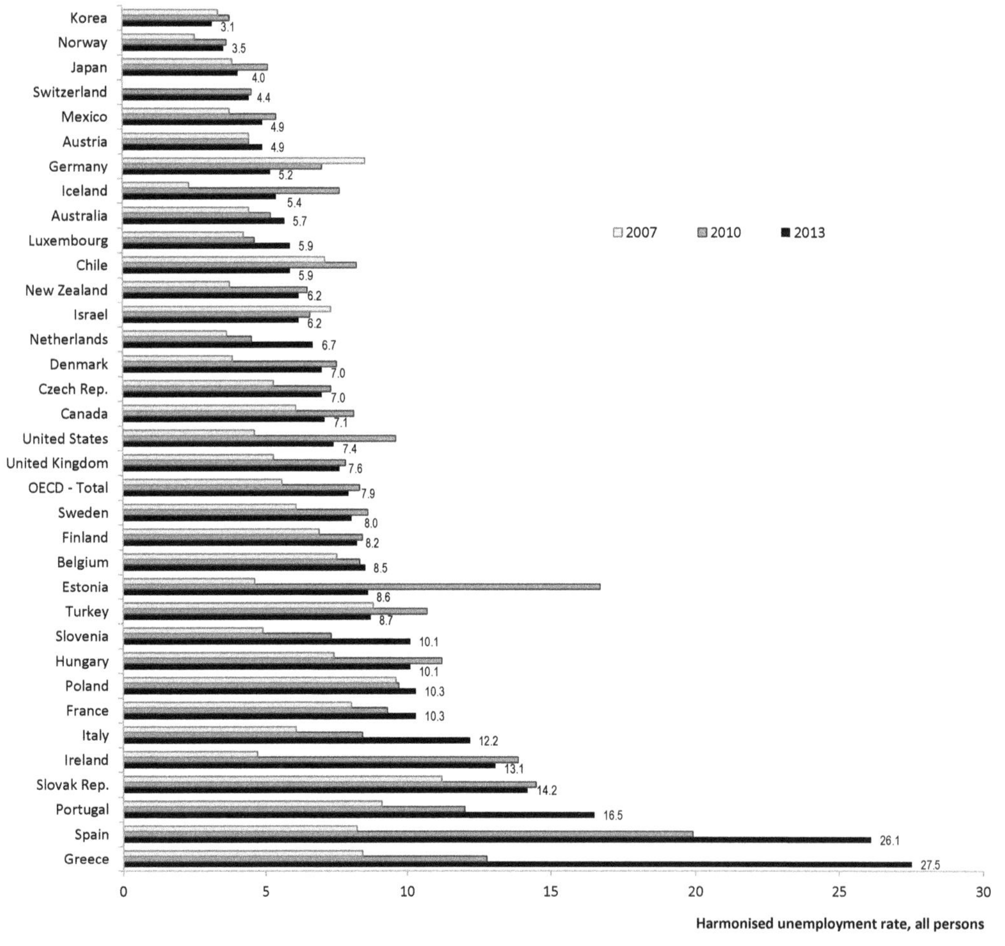

Source: ALFS (harmonised unemployment rate) (extracted from OECD.Stat in February 2015).

StatLink http://dx.doi.org/10.1787/888933325952

However, previous experiences with recessions show that employment in the health and social sector tends to be less sensitive to cyclical fluctuations than employment in other sectors. For example, in Canada, while total employment declined during the economic recessions of the early 1990s and in 2008-09, employment in the health and social sector continued to grow. The same holds true for the United States, France and Italy (Figure 2.3).

Figure 2.3. Employment in health and social sector compared with total employment, selected OECD countries, 1990 to 2014

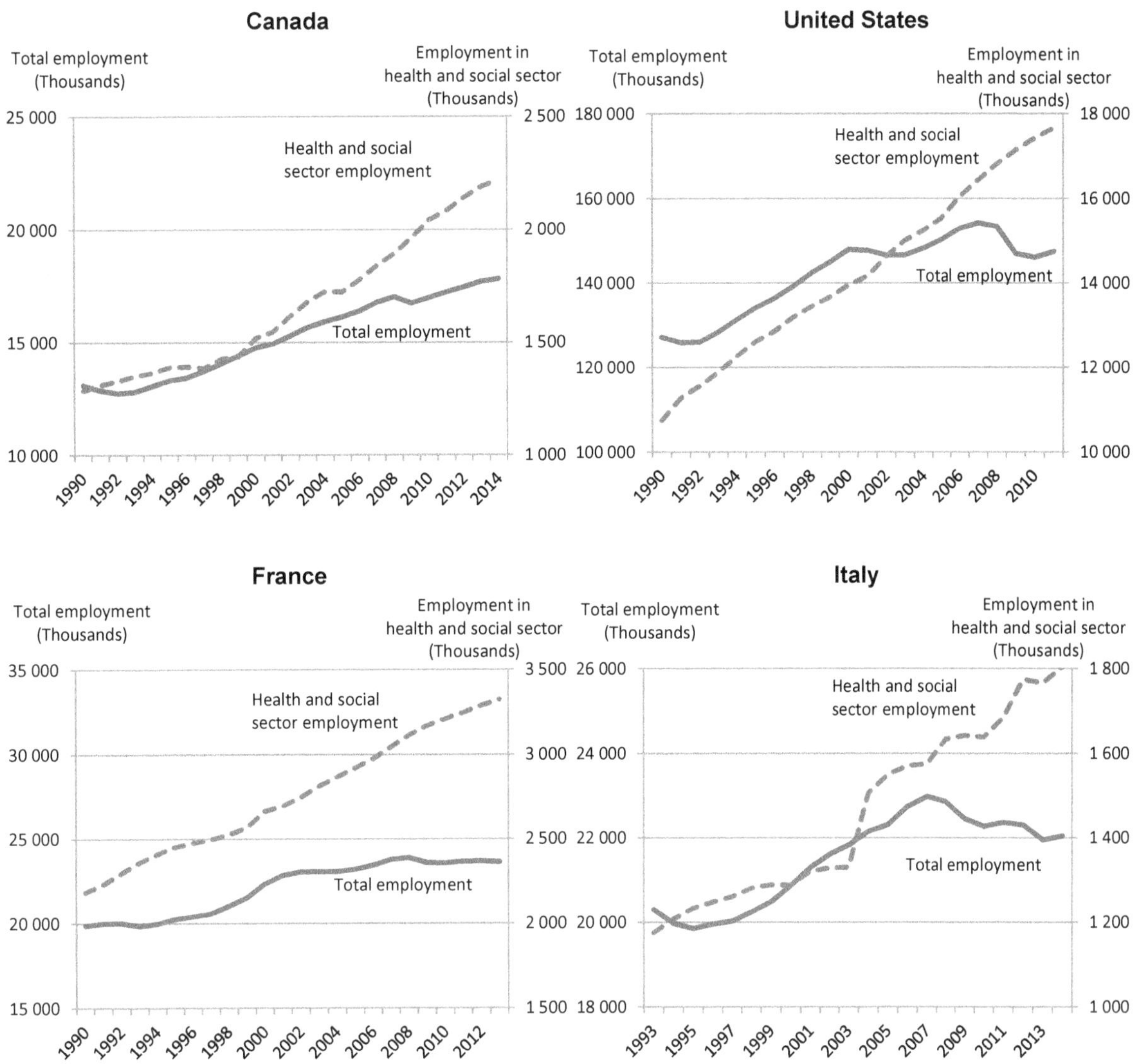

Source: For Canada, France and Italy: OECD.Stat, Annual Labour Force Survey (ALFS); for the United States: OECD.Stat, Structural Analysis (STAN) Database. All data extracted in January 2016.

StatLink http://dx.doi.org/10.1787/888933325968

Changes in employment of doctors and nurses in OECD countries

In 2013, the number of doctors and nurses was greater than in 2000 in nearly all OECD countries, both in absolute numbers and on a per capita basis. The economic crisis did not halt this rise, although it did curb the growth in some countries (Figures 2.4 and 2.5). The only OECD countries where the number of doctors per capita was not greater in 2013 than in 2000 were Israel (where the number of doctors grew less rapidly than the population since 2000) and France (where the number of doctors grew at the same pace as the population, so the density remained constant). For nurses, the only exceptions were Israel again (where the number of nurses also increased less rapidly than the population since 2000) and the Slovak Republic (where the number of nurses decreased during that period).

On average across OECD countries, the number of doctors increased from 2.7 doctors per 1 000 population in 2000 to 3.3 in 2013. The growth rate was particularly rapid in some countries which started with lower levels in 2000 (Turkey, Korea and Mexico), but also in countries which already had a large number in 2000 as is the case of Greece and Austria. In Greece though, most of this growth occurred before the economic crisis. In the United Kingdom, the number of doctors per capita increased by 40% between 2000 and 2013. Though initially driven by inflows of foreign-trained doctors, more recently the growth can be attributed to a larger number of domestic graduates.

Regarding nurses, the number increased from 7.8 per 1 000 population in 2000 to 9.1 in 2013 on average across OECD countries, an increase of 15% on a per capita basis during this whole period. The increase was particularly large in Switzerland, Norway and Denmark.

In 2013, there remained large differences in the number of doctors and nurses per capita across OECD countries, reflecting not only variations in overall health spending, but also in the organisation of health service delivery. With regards to doctors, the number ranged from less than two doctors per 1 000 population in Turkey and Chile, to over four per 1 000 population in Greece, Austria, Norway, Portugal and Germany, although the number in Portugal is over-estimated (as it includes all doctors licensed to practice). As for nurses, the number per capita was lowest in Turkey, Mexico and Greece, and highest in Switzerland, Norway, Denmark and Iceland.

Figure 2.4. Practising doctors per 1 000 population, OECD countries, 2000 and 2013 (or nearest year)

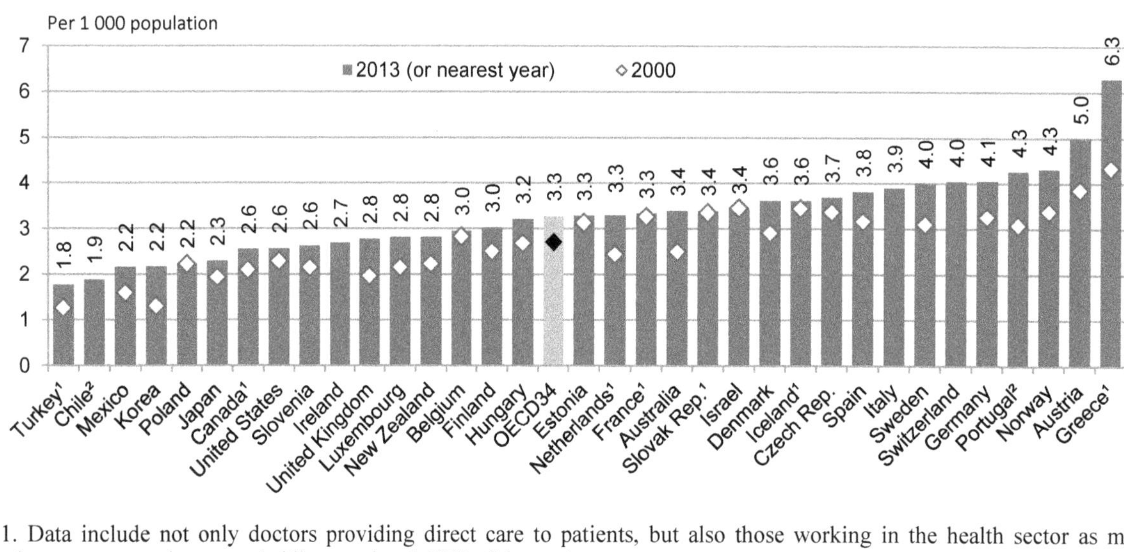

1. Data include not only doctors providing direct care to patients, but also those working in the health sector as managers, educators, researchers, etc. (adding another 5-10% of doctors).

2. Data refer to all doctors licensed to practice (resulting in a large over-estimation of the number of practising doctors in Portugal, of around 30%).

Source: OECD Health Statistics 2015.

StatLink http://dx.doi.org/10.1787/888933325971

Figure 2.5. Practising nurses per 1 000 population, OECD countries, 2000 and 2013 (or nearest year)

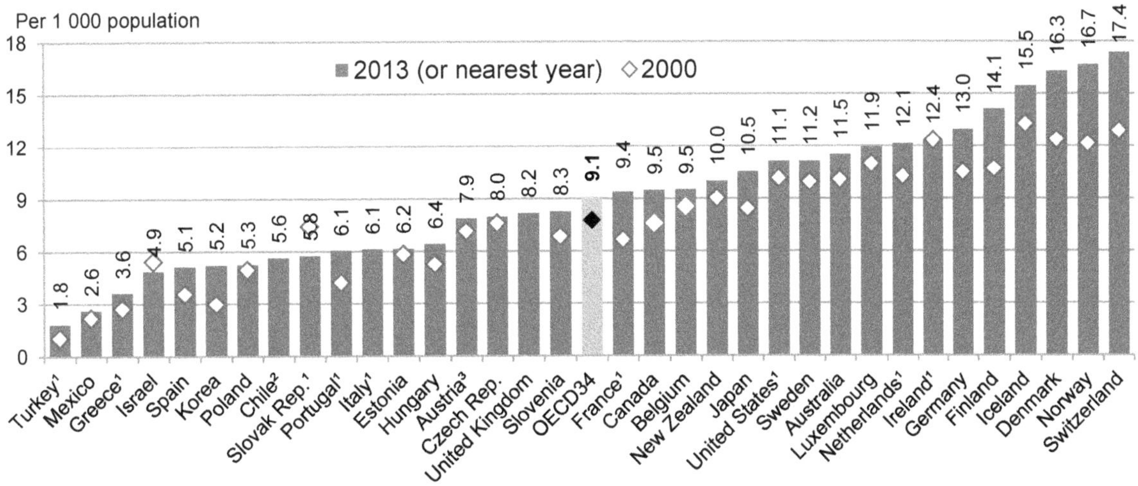

1. Data include not only nurses providing direct care to patients, but also those working in the health sector as managers, educators, researchers, etc.

2. Data in Chile refer to all nurses licensed to practice (less than one-third are professional nurses with a university degree).

3. Austria reports only nurses employed in hospital.

Source: OECD Health Statistics 2015.

StatLink http://dx.doi.org/10.1787/888933325986

The "skill mix" – as measured by the number of nurses per doctor – also differs widely across OECD countries. In many countries, there were between two to four nurses per doctor in 2013; yet, this ratio varied from less than one nurse per doctor in Greece to 4.5 nurses per doctor (or over) in Finland, Japan, Ireland and Denmark (Figure 2.6). These variations reflect different ways of organising health care delivery and the distribution of tasks among different health care providers. In Greece, the evidence suggests an oversupply of doctors and undersupply of nurses, resulting in an inefficient allocation of resources.

Figure 2.6. Ratio of nurses per physician, OECD countries, 2013 (or nearest year)

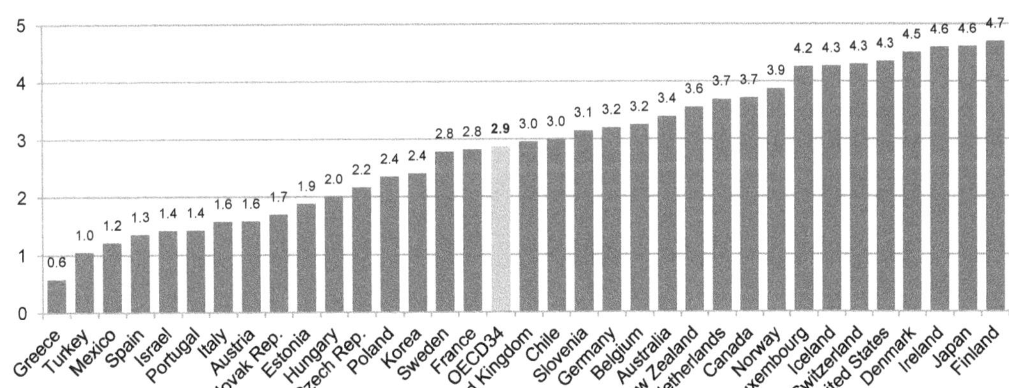

Source: OECD Health Statistics 2015.

StatLink http://dx.doi.org/10.1787/888933325992

Figure 2.7 looks more specifically at the growth in the absolute number of doctors and nurses employed in some OECD countries over the past decade (not taking into account the growth in population size).

Figure 2.7. Change in number of doctors and nurses, selected OECD countries, 2000 to 2014 (or nearest year)

Index (baseline year = 100)

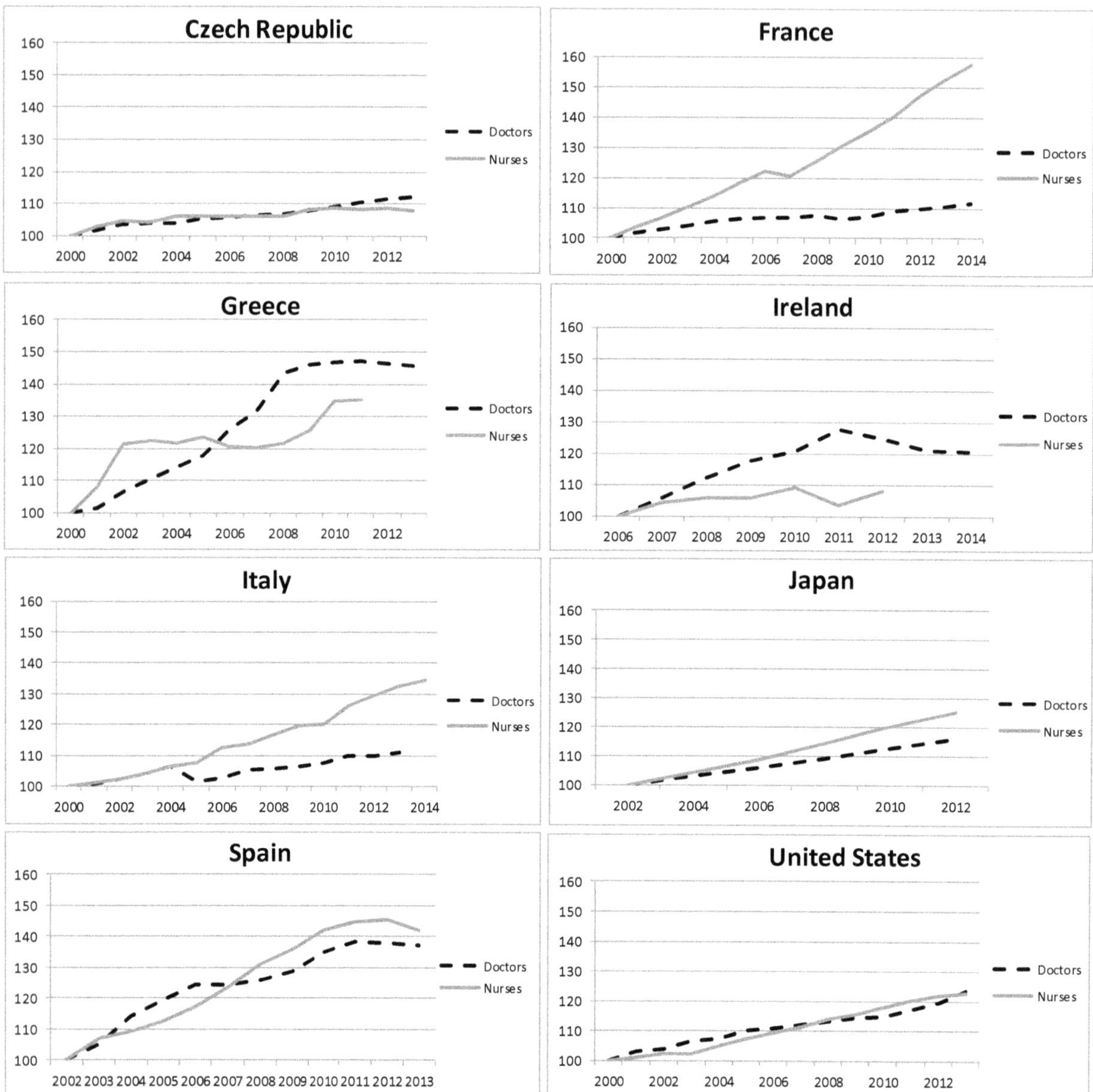

Source: OECD Health Statistics 2015.

StatLink http://dx.doi.org/10.1787/888933326009

In the United States, the absolute number of doctors and nurses has increased fairly steadily since 2000, rising from less than 700 000 doctors in 2000 to over 850 000 in 2013, and from less than 2 900 000 nurses in 2000 to over 3 500 000 in 2013. This growth has been driven mainly by an increase in the number of graduates from medicine and nursing (see Chapter 3) and a growing number of foreign-trained doctors and nurses (see Chapter 4).

In Japan and France, the number of doctors and nurses has also increased over the past decade, with the number of nurses growing much more rapidly (especially in France) than the number of doctors.

In Greece, the number of doctors increased strongly between 2000 and 2008, but has stabilised since then.

In Ireland, the number of doctors and nurses working in the health system has come down a few years following the economic crisis, but their number remains higher than before the crisis.

A few other European countries that have been hard hit by the recession have reduced temporarily the size of their health workforce. That is the case, for instance, of Estonia where the number of nurses employed was cut down in 2008, but the number has gone back up since then (not shown).

Changes in the remuneration of doctors and nurses

In many OECD countries, the economic crisis and the following marked slowdown or reduction in health spending had a greater impact on the remuneration of nurses and doctors than on their employment rate. Several European countries hard hit by the recession have notably cut down at least temporarily the wages or fees for doctors and nurses in efforts to reduce cost while protecting access to care for the population.

In Ireland, a series of measures from 2009 resulted not only in a freeze on recruitment and promotion, but also in actual cuts in wages of health care workers and lower fees paid to GPs (Morgan and Astolfi, 2014). Doctors in Denmark, Estonia, Italy and Slovenia also saw their salaries decreased in nominal terms in certain years after the crisis, and the same was also true for nurses in Estonia and Italy (Figure 2.8). In some other countries like the United Kingdom, the government imposed freezes for all public sector employees, including those working in the health sector.

In the most recent years, the salaries of doctors and nurses have started to go up again in several countries. This has been particularly the case in the Slovak Republic where doctors, nurses and other health workers obtained significant pay increases starting in 2012, following protests and emigration of a large number of doctors and nurses to other EU countries in previous years. Many doctors and nurses in Hungary were also granted a hefty pay raise starting in 2012 for the same reasons (see Section 4.6 in Chapter 4).

In Israel, a country that was hardly affected by the economic crisis, the salaries of doctors was increased significantly following an agreement in 2010 between the Israeli physician union and their employers.

Figure 2.8. Growth rate in the remuneration of doctors, nurses, and the average wage for all workers in the economy, in nominal terms, selected OECD countries, 2005 to 2014 (or nearest year)

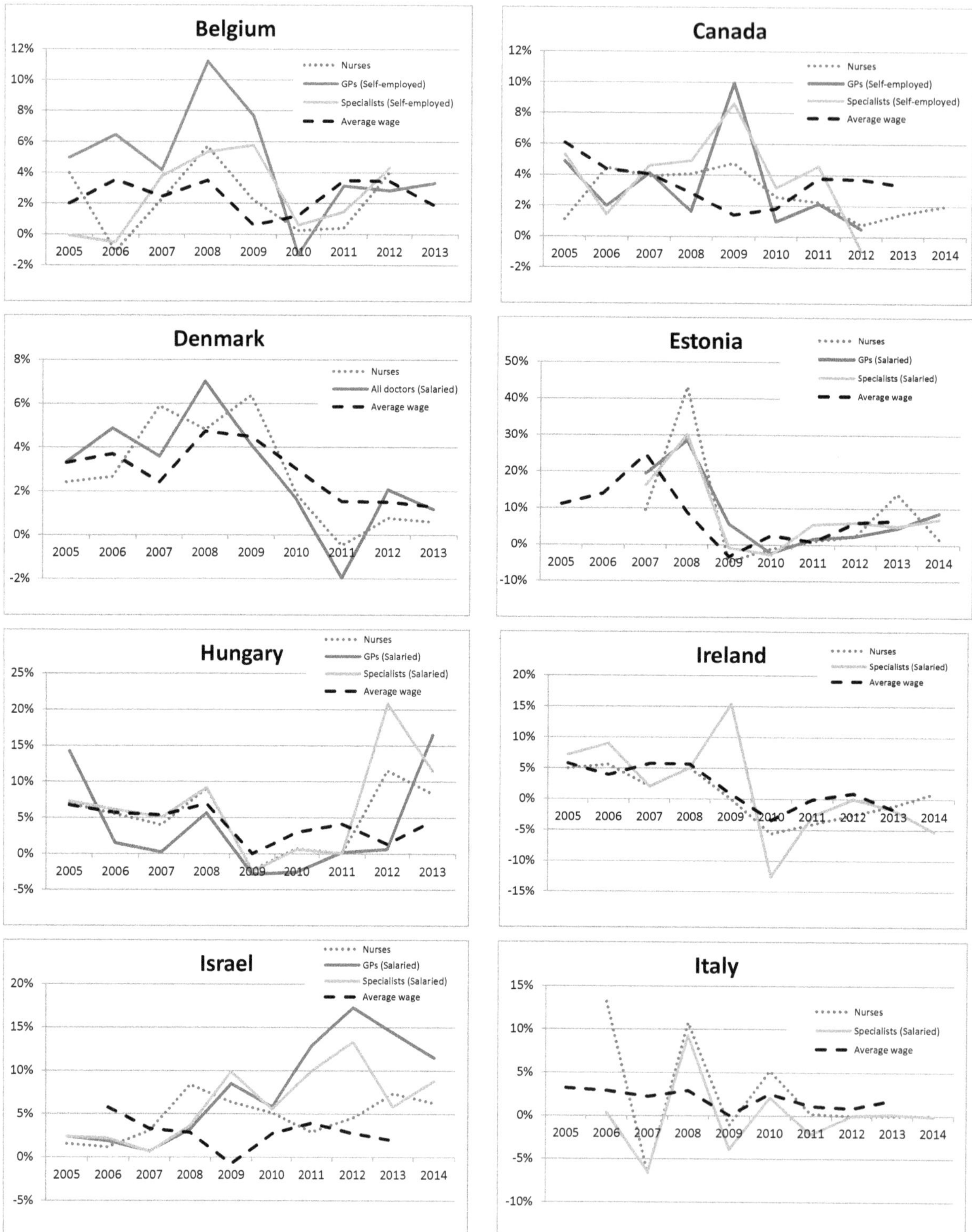

Figure 2.8. Growth rate in the remuneration of doctors, nurses, and the average wage for all workers in the economy, in nominal terms, selected OECD countries, 2005 to 2014 (or nearest year) *(cont.)*

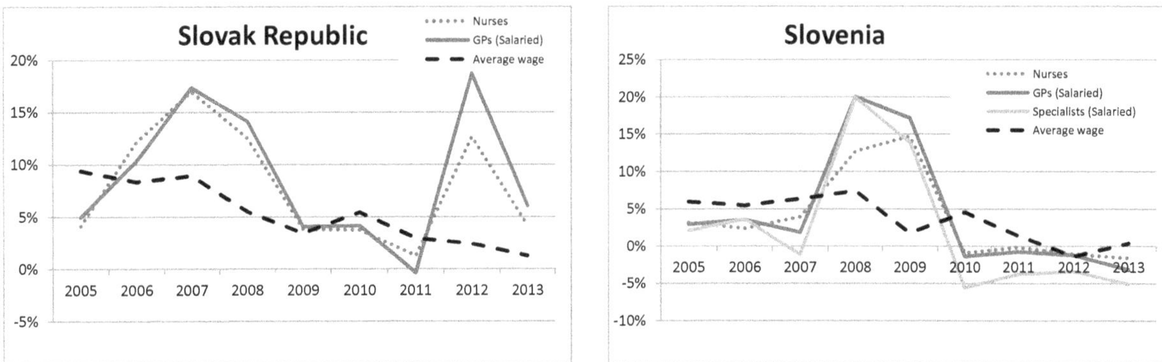

Note: All data refer to nominal wages (not adjusted for inflation).

Source: OECD Health Statistics 2015.

StatLink http://dx.doi.org/10.1787/888933326018

Prior to the economic downturn, several countries had signalled their intention to move to more flexible wage setting, at least within the hospital sector. But this intention does not seem to have been achieved in practice or in full for public sector hospitals in most countries. Fiscal pressures have led countries like France and the United Kingdom to "recentralise" their wage setting, as this appears to be perceived as an important regulatory tool for governments in times of fiscal constraint (Buchan et al., 2014).

2.3. Recent policy priorities on health workforce issues

Following the economic crisis, the budgetary context for health policy making changed quite radically in many OECD countries. In the years following the crisis, public and private spending on health either slowed down markedly or was cut down in several countries, reducing at least temporarily the demand for different categories of health workers. Combined with the fairly steady increase in the supply of health workers, this reduced concerns about widespread shortage of doctors, nurses and other health workers. Against this background, this section draws on responses from the *2012-13 OECD Health System Characteristics Survey* to describe some of the main health workforce priorities following the economic crisis as well as some of the actual policy responses.

The health workforce module in the *2012-13 OECD Health System Characteristics Survey* included five main questions on: 1) issues related to physician supply; 2) policies to address issues related to physician supply; 3) policies related to entry into medical education and training (so-called *numerus clausus*); 4) recent changes in medical and nursing student intakes; and 5) regulations of practice location. Most OECD countries (31 out of 34) responded to the survey, although not all answered all questions.

Out of the 31 OECD countries that responded to this Survey, only one country (the Netherlands) reported having no particular concern about physician supply. Among the other countries, five responded being concerned with the ability to maintain the overall supply of physicians (i.e., replacing those who are expected to retire in the years ahead). A slightly greater number of countries (nine) indicated that responding to a growing demand for physician services was a challenge. Twelve countries reported that they were struggling to maintain the share of general practitioners (GPs), while 23 countries reported having some shortages in certain specialty areas (although the medical specialties in question vary from one country to another and also within different regions in each country). The mal-distribution of doctors across different geographic regions was the most commonly reported concern, with 28 countries out of 31 reporting this as a challenge (Figure 2.9).[2]

Figure 2.9. Issues related to physician supply, OECD countries, 2012

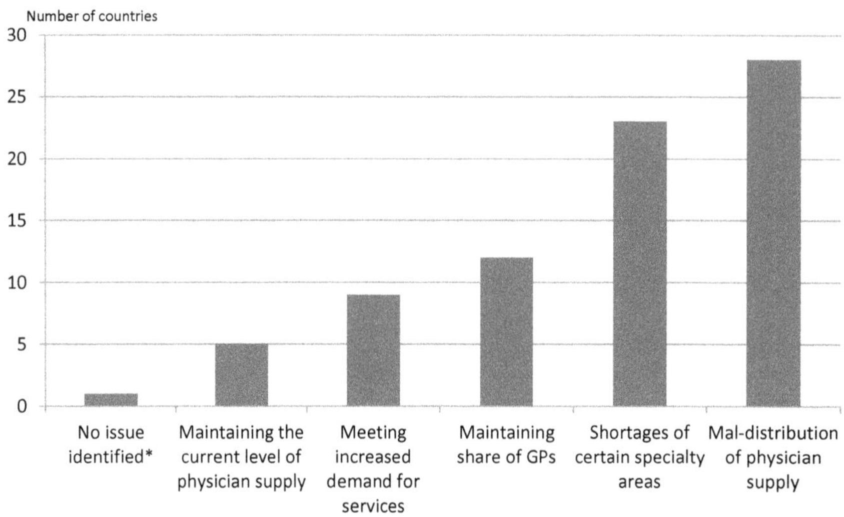

* The Netherlands is the only country that did not indicate any particular issue about physician supply.

Source: 2012-13 OECD Health System Characteristics Survey (based on 31 country responses).

StatLink http://dx.doi.org/10.1787/888933326024

OECD countries can use a range of policy levers to address issues related to physician supply. In the *2012-13 Health System Characteristics Survey*, countries were invited to indicate whether they had policies in place in seven areas. The responses to this survey (shown in Figure 2.10) indicate that:

- Five countries have policies to prolong the working lives of physicians, such as incentives for postponing retirement (the Czech Republic, France, Israel, Italy and Portugal);
- Six countries have targeted immigration policies to attract foreign physicians in the country, sometimes referring to specific underserved areas (Ireland, Israel, New Zealand, Portugal, Slovenia and the United States);
- Eleven countries are providing incentives (financial or non-financial) to encourage more doctors to choose general practice (Belgium, Canada, the Czech Republic, Germany, Hungary, Iceland, Luxembourg, Poland, Switzerland, the United Kingdom and the United States);
- Eleven countries are providing some incentives to foster the take-up of certain specialties that are deemed to be in shortages now or expected in the future (Canada, the Czech Republic, Denmark, Hungary, Iceland, Israel, Japan, New Zealand, Norway, Poland and the United States);

- Eleven countries have introduced or expanded the roles of non-physician providers to relieve pressures on physicians (Canada, Chile, Finland, Ireland, the Netherlands, New Zealand, Slovenia, Spain, Sweden, Switzerland and the United States);
- Sixteen countries have increased the overall intake into medical education and training;
- Eighteen countries indicated that they have put in place some financial incentives to correct a perceived geographic mal-distribution of physicians.

Figure 2.10. Policies in place to address identified physician supply problems, OECD countries, 2012

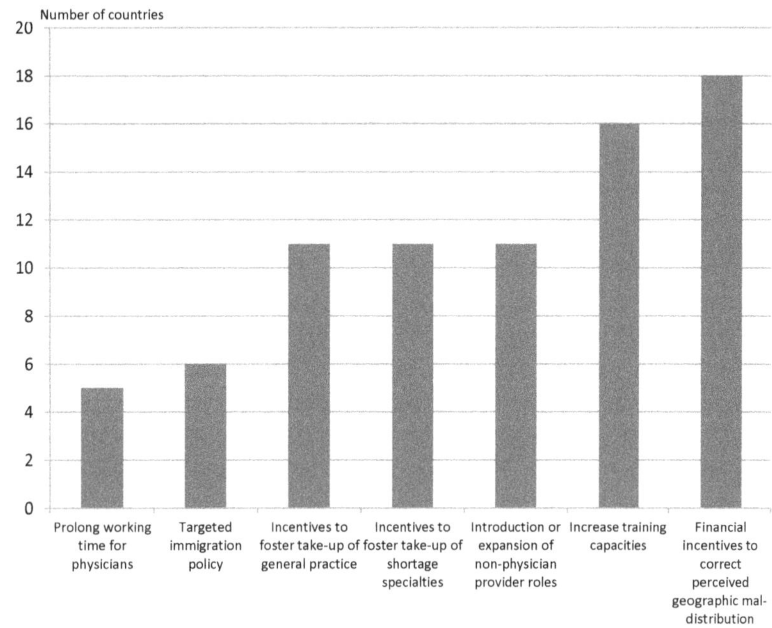

Source: 2012-13 OECD Health System Characteristics Survey (based on 31 country responses).

StatLink http://dx.doi.org/10.1787/888933326039

The following sections of this chapter focus on policies that different OECD countries have adopted: 1) to increase the retention rates and the retirement age of doctors and nurses to maintain or increase supply; 2) to achieve a better balance between general practitioners and specialists (and also between different specialties) to respond to changing health care needs; and 3) to expand the roles for non-physicians to improve access to care and reduce the demand for doctors. Chapter 3 describes recent changes in policies concerning student intakes in medical and nursing education programmes (one of the main policy levers to adjust the future supply of doctors and nurses), while Chapter 4 reviews the range of policies that different OECD countries have put in place to promote a more even geographic distribution of doctors and health services.

Increasing retention rates and retirement age of doctors and nurses

This section reviews recent trends in the retention rates of nurses and the retirement patterns of doctors and nurses, and describes how various policies might have affected these trends.

Increasing the retention rates of nurses throughout their working life continues to be an important issue in many OECD countries, as many leave the profession well before the standard retirement age. A large number of nurses leave very shortly after their entry into the profession (e.g., some leave, at least temporarily, during their pregnancy and to raise their children), while a large number leaves a few years before the standard retirement age. For example, in Canada, the exit rates of registered nurses (RNs) in 2007 (that is, just before the economic crisis of 2008-09) was estimated to be 6% per year for those aged 25-34, 2% for those aged 35-49, 3% for those aged 50-59, and 11% for those aged 60-64 (Canadian Nurses Association, 2009).

As has been observed in previous recessions, there is evidence in many countries that the recent economic downturn has increased the retention rates of nurses and also led to the re-entry of a certain number of nurses who had previously left their occupation. In the United States, a significant number of job vacancies right after the onset of the recession were filled by nurses who had previously left their jobs (Buerhaus et al., 2009). In Australia, the exit rates of nurses in 2007 and 2008 were much lower than in previous years, at least partly explained by the economic crisis and its impact on labour market conditions.

In its 2012 projections of the future supply of registered nurses (RNs) in Australia, Health Workforce Australia used two different assumptions regarding future retention rates: the first assumption (under the main scenario) was that the exit rates would return to their pre-crisis levels by 2012 (that is, around 5% to 6% per year), while the second assumption (under the alternative scenario) was that they would remain at their lower levels of 2007-08 over the entire projection period (i.e., around 2% per year). These two different assumptions led to very different results in terms of the projected shortage of RNs in the years ahead. While the baseline scenario estimated a possible shortage of 80 000 nurses in Australia by 2025, the shortage would come down to only 15 000 nurses if the exit rates remained at their 2007-08 levels throughout the projection period (Figure 2.11).

In some countries, various policies and programmes have been adopted to promote greater retention rates of nurses in the profession. In many cases, the adoption of these initiatives preceded the economic crisis, but some of these initiatives have been pursued in recent years, possibly also contributing to higher retention rates. In Australia, several nurse retention initiatives offer opportunities for career development, through a range of programmes providing nurses with financial support and time off to pursue those activities (Department of Health, 2013). In other countries, nurses have obtained substantial pay increases as an incentive to keep working. This has been the case in a few Central and Eastern European countries which were confronted with substantial exit rates, as nurses moved to other European countries offering better pay rates (see Chapter 4 in this publication for more information on these policies).

Figure 2.11. Projected demand and supply of registered nurses based on two alternative scenarios about exit rates, Australia, 2009 to 2025

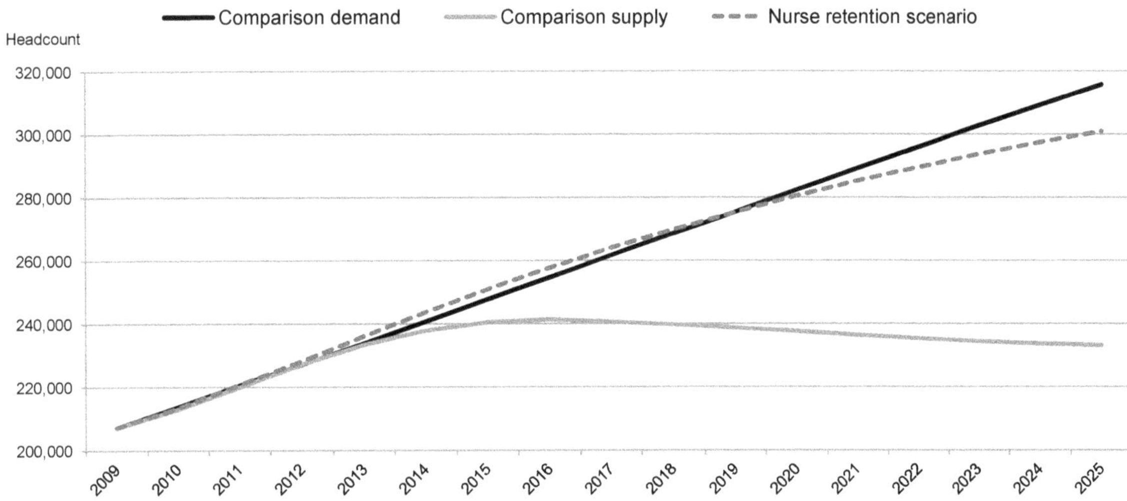

Note: The "comparison supply" projections are based on the assumption that the exit rates would return to its higher level prior to 2007-08, while the "scenario supply" is based on the assumption that they would remain at the same (lower) level of 2007-08.

Source: Health Workforce Australia (2012), *Health Workforce 2025 – Doctors, Nurses and Midwives: Vol. 1 and Vol. 2.*

StatLink http://dx.doi.org/10.1787/888933326046

On average across OECD countries, nearly one in three doctors (33%) were 55 years or older in 2013, up from around one in five (21%) in 2000. The percentage of doctors aged 55 and over is much higher than the share of all workers in the economy in this age group (19% on average in 2013). However, the proportion of doctors aged 55 and over varies considerably across countries, ranging from only about 13% in the United Kingdom to 45% or more in Israel, Italy and France (Figure 2.12). In the coming years, many countries will face the challenge of replacing the large number of doctors who will retire, although the size and timing of these replacement needs will largely depend on their retirement patterns.

The share of nurses aged 55 and over has also increased in many OECD countries. For example, in Australia, France and the United States, more than 20% of nurses were aged 55 and over in 2013 (or most recent year available), up from around 10% only in 2000 (Figure 2.13).

Pension reforms, as well as a possible greater willingness and capacity of many doctors and nurses to work longer, are likely to have a significant impact on future replacement needs.

Figure 2.12. Share of doctors aged over 55 as a percentage of all doctors, selected OECD countries, 2000 to 2013

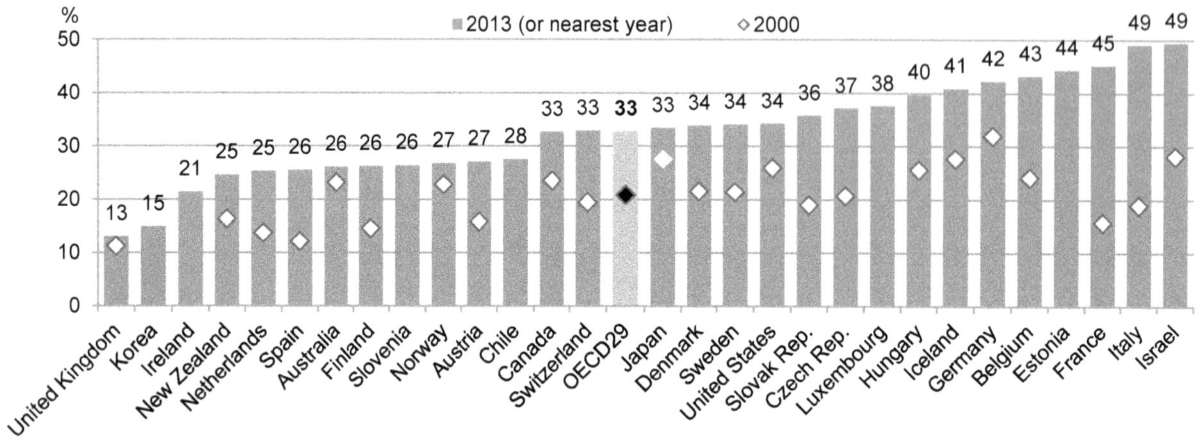

Source: OECD Health Statistics 2015.

StatLink http://dx.doi.org/10.1787/888933326057

Figure 2.13. Share of nurses in different age categories, selected OECD countries, 2000 to 2013 (or nearest year)

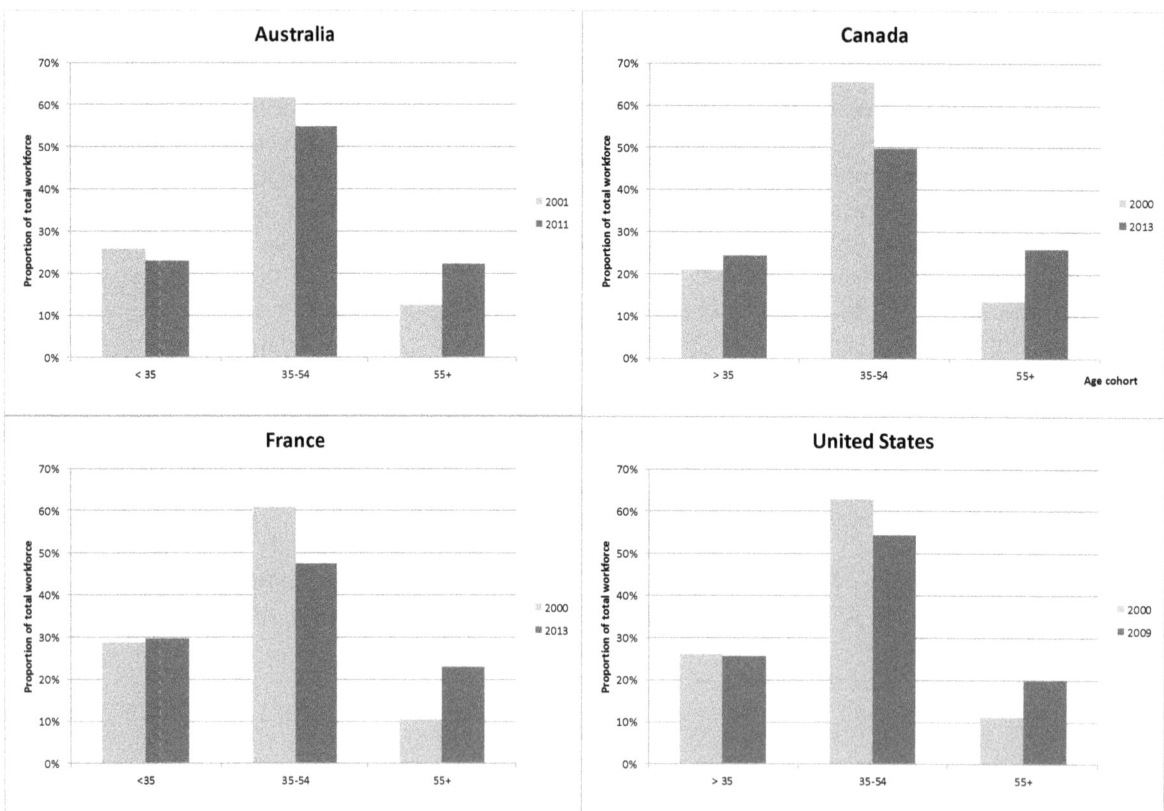

Source: Australia: Review of Australian Government Health Workforce Programs, 2013. Canada: Health Workforce Database (CIHI). France: DRESS. United States: The U.S. Nursing Workforce: Trends in Supply and Education (HRSA).

StatLink http://dx.doi.org/10.1787/888933326060

Several OECD countries have reformed their pension systems and increased the retirement age to take into account longer life expectancy. According to the *OECD Pensions Outlook 2014*, the overall retirement age is being raised in an increasing number of OECD countries, often beyond 65 which has generally been the norm in most countries for the past decade (OECD, 2014b). While there are few studies examining the impact of these pension reforms specifically on health workers, it is likely that these reforms will prolong their working lives and expand the supply of doctors and nurses after age 65 in the coming years.

Five countries (the Czech Republic, France, Israel, Italy and Portugal) indicated that part of their strategies to try to maintain or increase the supply of doctors is to prolong their working lives, either through general pension policy reforms increasing the retirement age of all workers or through more specific incentives for doctors to postpone their retirement. As recent developments in some countries show, physicians may also choose to delay their retirement for other reasons, for instance, due to unexpected losses in investment value of retirement plans following the financial and economic crisis or difficulties in selling their practice. It is not always clear whether the recent increase in the effective retirement age of doctors in some countries is due to cyclical factors only (which may be temporary) or reflects the impact of more structural factors (e.g., longer life expectancy) or structural policies (increase in retirement age).

The impact on the supply of physicians of any postponement in the retirement age can be very significant. In France, recent increases in the participation rate of doctors beyond 65 have been the main driver of the overall increase in the number of doctors since 2008 (see Box 2.1).

Box 2.1. Recent findings on work-to-retirement transitions of doctors

The Canadian Institute for Health Information released a report in 2011 on the work-to-retirement transitions of doctors in Canada. This report used information from a number of data sources to determine the scope of activities of doctors around retirement age (Pong, 2011). One of its main conclusions was that the assumption of a fixed retirement age (e.g. at age 65) is increasingly unrealistic, as the activities of many physicians go well beyond that age, albeit often combined with a gradual reduction in their working hours (rather than a sudden and complete exit from the labour force).

In the Netherlands, the Advisory Committee on Medical Manpower Planning (ACMMP) regularly conducts scenario-based projection exercises to advise the government and other key stakeholders on the number of students who should be admitted in initial medical education and the number of graduates who should be admitted to different specialty training. As part of the 2013 projection exercise, the ACMMP commissioned a report to look at recent trends in physician retirement patterns observed during the economic crisis (Van der Windt, 2013). The report examined at what age doctors in the Netherlands retired fully and how this has changed in recent years. It found that the effective retirement age of doctors in the Netherlands has increased by 1.5 years (from 61 to 62.5 years) in a period of two years only, between 2008 and 2010 (Van der Windt, 2013). This report was not able to provide definitive explanations for this rapid increase, but suggested that an important factor might be the impact of the economic downturn, especially for self-employed doctors whose retirement funds may have lost value during the financial crisis. However, the report did not rule out that structural and lasting factors might also have contributed to this increase in retirement age.

In France also, there is growing evidence that the retirement patterns of doctors are evolving, with the effective retirement age increasing significantly. Most of the increase in the number of doctors in France since 2008 is due to a growing number of doctors working beyond the age of 65 (DREES, 2014). The speed and scale of this development was unexpected in a projection exercise that was carried out by the Ministry of Health in 2009 using data prior to 2008 as the baseline, although one of the alternative scenarios estimated the impact of a possible postponement in their retirement age (Attal-Toubert and Vanderschelden, 2009).

The use of more flexible and realistic assumptions about the retirement patterns of doctors in projection models is important to assess more precisely future replacement needs. Some health workforce planning models have achieved progress in this direction. For example, in the Netherlands, the model used by the Advisory Committee on Medical Manpower Planning takes into account that some doctors continue to practice beyond the standard retirement age in their estimation of exit rates (ACMMP, 2010; 2014). In France, the 2009 physician projection model of the Ministry of Health included a scenario assuming a two year postponement of the effective retirement age of doctors (phased in over a five-year period). This assumption had a considerable impact on the projected supply: the total number of doctors was estimated to grow by 4% from 2006 to 2030, compared to a 1% decline over the same period in the "status quo" scenario (Attal-Toubert and Vanderschelden, 2009).

Similarly, the results from the 2011 projections of the future supply of nurses in France estimated that the 2010 pension reforms might increase the number of active nurses by 3.5% by 2030, compared with a "status quo" scenario (Barlet and Cavillon, 2011).

Achieving a better balance between generalists and specialists, and the mix of specialties

OECD countries differ significantly in the composition of their physician workforce, notably in the balance between medical generalists and specialists. Such differences reflect different ways of organising health service delivery, allocating resources for specialty training, as well as the relative attractiveness of general medicine compared to other specialties.

Many countries have expressed concerns about the ability to maintain, if not increase, the number and share of general practitioners, in a context of ageing populations and a growing number of people living with one or more chronic conditions. Over the past two decades, the share of generalists (including general practitioners/family doctors and other generalists) has declined in most OECD countries. Between 1995 and 2014, their share decreased from 51% to 42% in Germany and from 35% to less than 30% in the United Kingdom, with most of the reduction occurring between 1995 and 2005. On average across OECD countries, only one-third of doctors are generalists nowadays (Figure 2.14).

In nearly all OECD countries, general practitioners earn much less than specialists. On average across OECD countries, general practitioners earn about 2.5 times the average wage of all workers in their countries, whereas specialists earn more than three times the average wage (OECD, 2015). In most countries, the remuneration gap between generalists and specialists has continued to widen in recent years, but there are some exceptions. In Austria, Belgium and the Netherlands, the growth in the remuneration of GPs has exceeded that of specialists, thereby narrowing the remuneration gap to some extent (Figure 2.15).

Figure 2.14. Generalists as a share of all physicians, selected OECD countries, 1995 to 2014 (or nearest year)

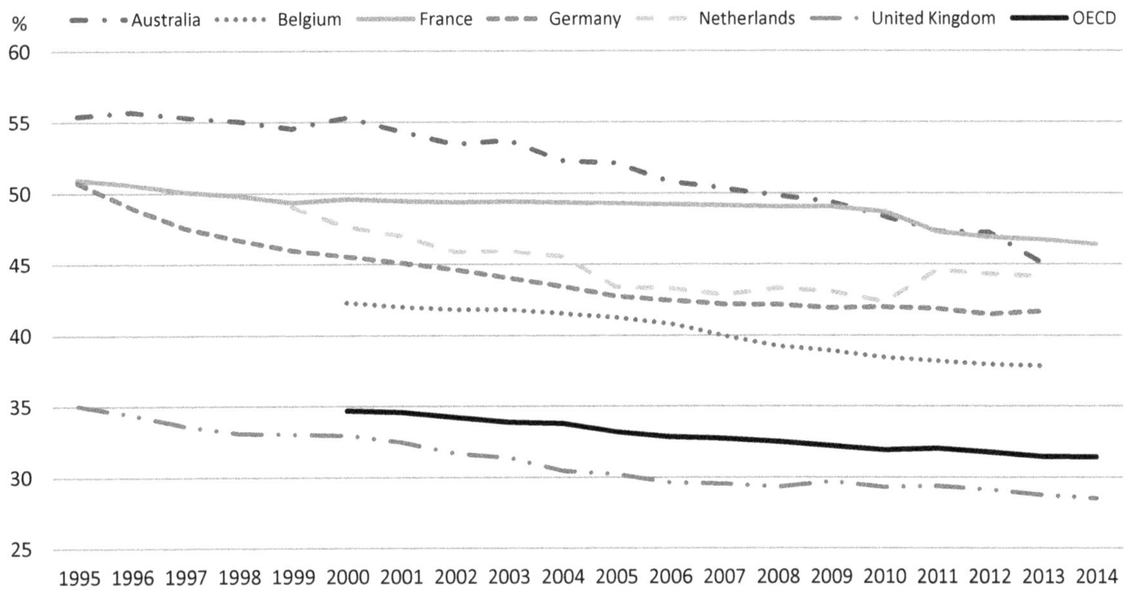

Note: Generalists include general practitioners ('family doctors') and other generalists (non-specialists).

Source: OECD Health Statistics 2015.

StatLink http://dx.doi.org/10.1787/888933326070

Figure 2.15. Growth in the remuneration of GPs and specialists, selected OECD countries, 2005 to 2013 (or nearest year)

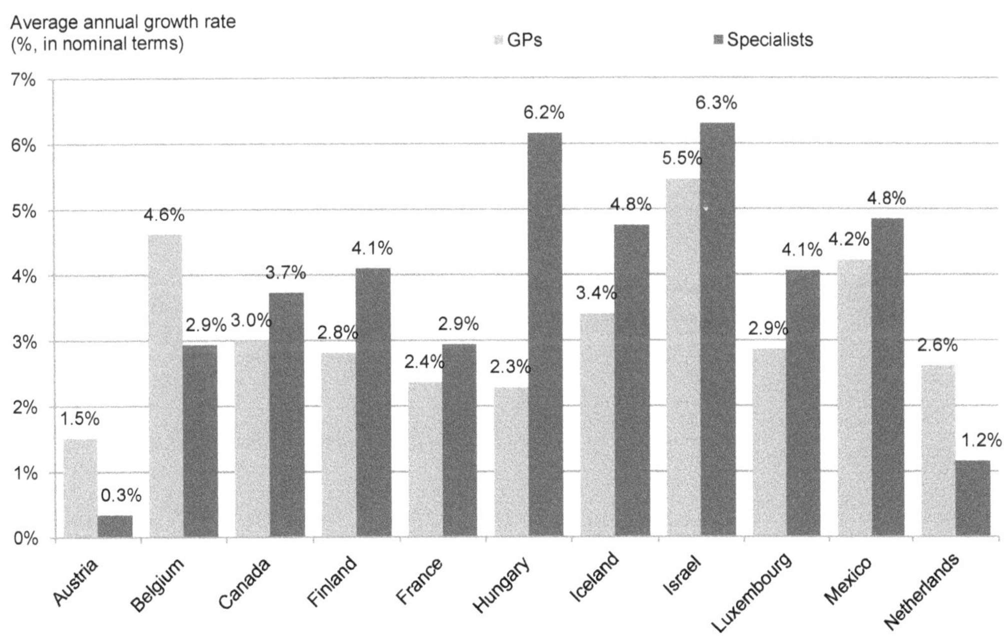

Source: OECD Health Statistics 2015.

StatLink http://dx.doi.org/10.1787/888933326080

Many OECD countries have introduced in recent years different programmes and incentives to encourage more students to choose general medicine with a view to strengthen their primary care system (Belgium, Canada, the Czech Republic, France, Germany, Hungary, Iceland, Luxembourg, Poland, Switzerland, the United Kingdom and the United States). One of the main measures has been to increase the number of post-graduate training places in general medicine (see Section 3.5 in Chapter 3 for further information on the experience in countries like France and Canada).

However, it is not sufficient to adjust the number of post-graduate training places to achieve a better mix of doctors. The allocation of training posts needs to be followed up by measures that make working conditions in general practice relatively attractive compared with other specialties, in order to avoid further specialisation and professional mobility. These measures include, for instance, reducing the remuneration gaps and reducing working time constraints often associated with general practice.

Many countries also have concerns about imbalances among different specialties. For example, in Canada, there are concerns that too many paediatricians are being trained, while the training of geriatricians and other doctors specialising in the care of elderly people remain very low (Figure 2.16).

Figure 2.16. Enrolment in post-graduate training in paediatrics and geriatric medicine, Canada, 2001-12

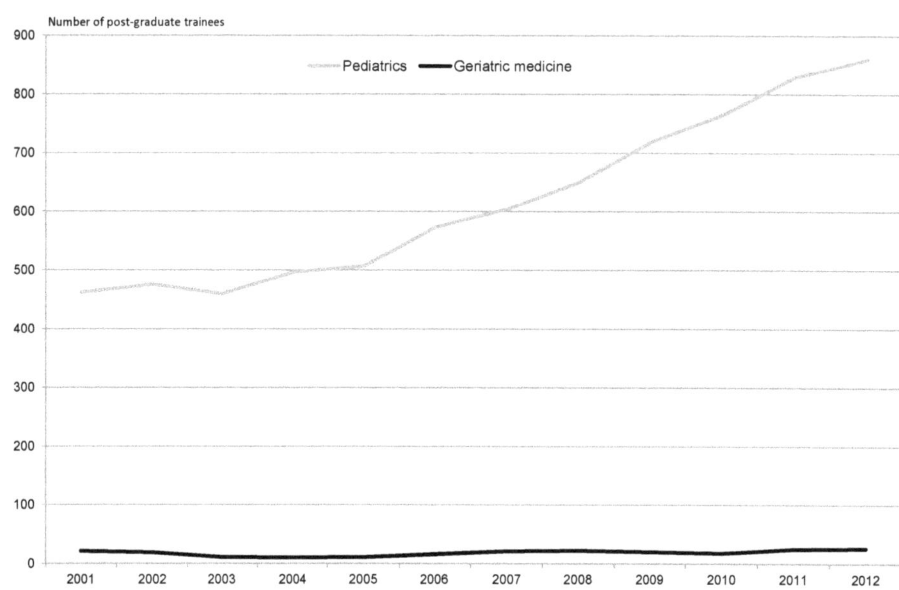

Source: CAPER (2014), database available at http://www.caper.ca.

StatLink http://dx.doi.org/10.1787/888933326097

Eleven countries indicated having policies in place to promote the choice of certain specialties which are deemed to be in shortage now or in the future (Canada, the Czech Republic, Denmark, Hungary, Iceland, Israel, Japan, New Zealand, Norway, Poland and the United States).

Expanding the roles for non-physicians

To counter potential shortages in physician supply, eleven countries responded to the *2012-13 OECD Health System Characteristics Survey* that they had introduced or expanded the role of non-physician providers over the past few years.

A 2010 OECD study documented the state of development of advanced roles for nurses in 12 OECD countries, focussing in particular on nurse practitioners (NPs) (Delamaire and Lafortune, 2010). Some countries, such as the United States, Canada and the United Kingdom, have established the role of NPs several decades ago. They often started in rural and remote areas where there were fewer doctors, and their roles and practice locations have expanded over time. The development of advanced practice nurses and NPs has been somewhat more recent in other countries such as Australia and Ireland. In other countries such as Belgium and France, the formal recognition of advanced practice nursing is still in its infancy; nonetheless, a number of pilot studies have been carried out in recent years to test new and more advanced roles, in some cases accompanied by a formal recognition of these roles.

Nurse practitioners (NPs) often practice in primary care and provide a set of services that might otherwise be performed by doctors (e.g., being the first contact for people with minor illness, providing routine follow-up of patients with chronic conditions, prescribing certain drugs and ordering tests). In many countries (mainly Anglo-Saxon countries: Australia, Canada, Ireland, the United Kingdom and the United States), NPs and other categories of nurses are now authorised to prescribe certain pharmaceutical drugs, with the list usually growing over time. The United States was the first country to introduce the right for nurses to prescribe drugs in the mid-1970s, followed by the United Kingdom and Australia at the beginning of the 1990s. In Canada, ten out of the 13 jurisdictions now allow NPs to prescribe controlled drugs and substances independently. Ireland started to authorise this type of practice in 2007. In all of these countries, the authorisation for nurses to prescribe medications has required legislative changes (Delamaire and Lafortune, 2010).

An important distinction regarding the rights for nurses to prescribe drugs is whether they can prescribe independently or only under the supervision of a doctor. Some countries, such as the United States, have granted the authorisation for all advanced practice nurses to prescribe drugs, while others have been more restrictive and have granted it to some categories only. For instance, in Canada, only NPs in primary care are allowed to prescribe drugs without supervision by doctors. In some countries, such as the United Kingdom and Ireland, this authorisation may be granted to all nurses, provided they complete appropriate training. The range of drugs that nurses can prescribe in these countries is broad, including antibiotics, antiviral drugs, anticoagulants, anticholesterols and others. Nevertheless, there are variations across countries concerning the right for nurses to prescribe controlled drugs in particular (e.g., narcotics and strong pain killers).

Even in those countries that have the longest experience with establishing a nurse practitioner role, their number continues to be fairly limited and they only account for a small proportion of all nurses. In the United States, NPs represented 4.3% of the total number of RNs in 2013 (Bureau of Labor Statistics, 2013). In Canada, they accounted for an even smaller share, representing only 1.3% of all RNs in 2013, although their number and share have increased over the past decade (CIHI, 2014).

In the United States, over the past decade, the number of new graduates from training programmes for mid-level providers, such as physician assistants and NPs has been growing faster than that of medical graduates (Figure 2.17). It can therefore be expected that their relative importance will continue to grow in the years ahead.

Figure 2.17. Physician assistants, nurse practitioners and medical doctors' graduates, United States, 2000 to 2010

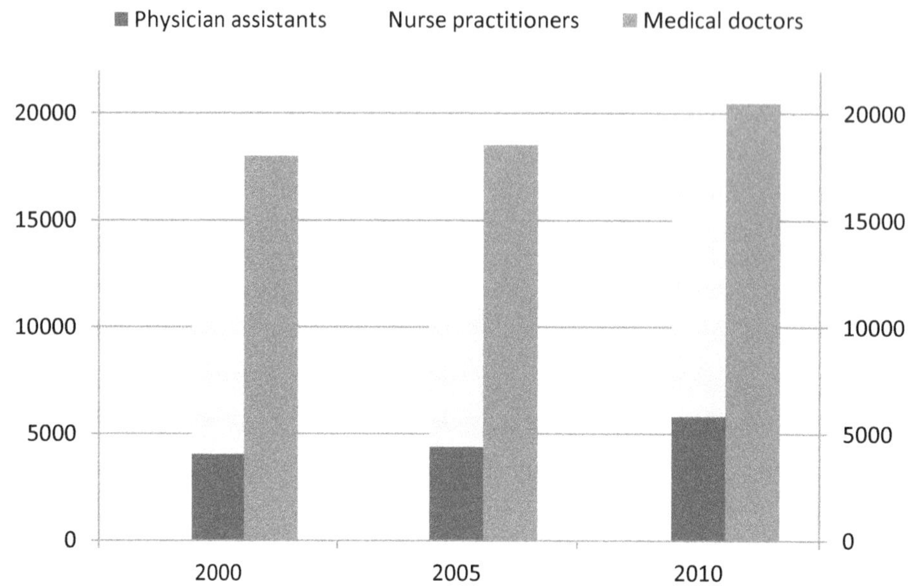

Source: OECD Health Statistics 2013, US National Commission on Certification of Physician Assistants "Certified Physician Assistant Population Trends (PA-Cs)", American Association of Colleges of Nursing 2000-2010 Annual Surveys.

StatLink http://dx.doi.org/10.1787/888933326109

In the Netherlands and Switzerland, health workforce projection models assume that such mid-level providers may be able to take on part of the services traditionally provided by GPs. In Switzerland, it has been estimated that promoting greater task substitution between GPs and NPs may lead to a slowdown in the number of GP consultations. This projection suggests that, between 2005 and 2030, GP consultations would only increase by 2% when there is task substitution, compared with a cumulative rise of 13% in a scenario assuming no substitution (Seematter-Bagnoud et al., 2007). In the Netherlands, the 2010 physician projection models estimated that a re-allocation of tasks from GPs to NPs may reduce the demand for GPs by 0.6% to 1.2% per year (ACMMP, 2010).

2.4. Conclusions

Over the past few years, a number of cyclical and structural factors have contributed to lessen concerns over a possible looming crisis in the health workforce in OECD countries. On the demand side, the economic crisis led to a marked slowdown or reduction in private and public spending on health, thereby also gradually reducing the demand for different categories of health workers. On the supply side, decisions to increase the number of students admitted in medical and nursing schools have resulted in growing numbers of new domestically-trained doctors and nurses entering the labour market. In some countries, these growing numbers of new domestic graduates have been accompanied by continued inflows of foreign-trained doctors and nurses.

In recent years, most OECD countries have experienced a substantial increase in health workers' retention rates, with a higher proportion of nurses remaining in the profession than in the past and a growing number of doctors continuing to practice beyond the traditional retirement age. In the case of nurses, this seems to be more related to the deterioration in general labour market conditions after the economic crisis and the lack of good alternative employment, rather than to any deliberate policies and programmes to improve their working conditions. Still, in some countries, some measures have been taken to encourage greater retention rates of nurses, including through increasing support for their continuous professional development and pay raise. As for physicians, the postponement of retirement age seems to be related to both cyclical and structural factors. The decline in asset values following the economic crisis has pushed some physicians to work longer in some countries. In addition, the deferral of retirement for both doctors and nurses is at least partly related to the impact of pension reforms, which have reduced incentives to take early retirement and increased the retirement age (or length of the contribution period).

Across OECD countries, population ageing and a growing number of people living with chronic diseases is expanding the demand for primary care to avoid unnecessary hospitalisation. But at the same time, the share of general practitioners in the medical workforce has declined in many OECD countries, due to a growing remuneration gap with specialists and greater working time constraints. To avoid shortages of general practitioners, a number of countries have decided to increase significantly the number of postgraduate training places in general medicine vis-à-vis other specialisations. But the success of this measure will also depend on the implementation of other complementary measures that will make general practice a more attractive career option for newly-trained doctors.

Over the past few years, many countries have also introduced or expanded the roles of non-physicians in primary care, such as nurse practitioners or pharmacists, to improve access to services and achieve efficiency gains. The experience in various countries shows that the introduction or expansion of these roles often needs to overcome the initial opposition from medical professionals, who may perceive these role extensions as a threat to their activity or a loss of quality for their patients. Nonetheless, several evaluations show that advanced practice nurses are able to deliver the same quality of care as doctors for a range of patients, including those with minor illnesses and those requiring routine follow-up, provided that they have acquired the required education and training. The opportunity to expand further the scope of practice of non-physicians will depend, to a certain extent, on the future supply and attitudes of physicians. Past experience shows that such extensions in scope of practice tend to be easier to implement in times and places where there are fewer physicians.

Notes

1. The authors are thankful to Frédéric Daniel (OECD) for statistical assistance.

2. The term "mal-distribution" of doctors is used here to describe an uneven number of doctors per capita across different regions. It is *not* used to describe issues related to the composition of the medical workforce (i.e., the mix between generalists and specialists, and the mix of different specialties).

References

ACMMP – Dutch Advisory Committee on Medical Manpower Planning (2014), *The 2013 Recommendations for Medical Specialist Training*, Capaciteitsogaan, Utrecht.

ACMMP (2010), *Capacity Plan, Vol. 2: General Medicine*, Capaciteitsplan, Utrecht.

Attal-Toubert, K. and M. Vanderschelden (2009), "La démographie médicale à l'horizon 2030: De nouvelles projections nationales et régionales détaillées", *Dossiers Solidarité Santé,* No. 12, DREES, Paris.

Barlet, M. and M. Cavillon (2011), "La démographie des infirmiers à l'horizon 2030", *Etudes et résultats*, No. 760, DREES, Paris.

Buchan, J., A. Kumar and M. Schoenstein (2014), "Wage-setting in the Hospital Sector", *OECD Health Working Papers No.77*, OECD Publishing, Paris, http://dx.doi.org/10.1787/5jxx56b8hqhl-en.

Buerhaus, P.I., D.I. Auerbach and D.O. Staiger (2009), "The Recent Surge In Nurse Employment: Causes And Implications", *Health Affairs*, Vol. 28, No. 4, pp. w657-w668, July/August.

Bureau of Labor Statistics (2013), *Occupational Employment Statistics*, May.

CIHI – Canadian Institute for Health Information (2014), *Regulated Nurses, 2013*, Ottawa, Canada.

CNA – Canadian Nurses Association (2009), *Tested Solutions for Eliminating Canada's Registered Nurse Shortage*, Report prepared by G. Tomblin Murphy et al., Canadian Nurses Association, Ottawa, http://www.nursesunions.ca/sites/default/files/rn_shortage_report_e.pdf.

Delamaire, M. and G. Lafortune (2010), "Nurses in Advanced Roles: A Description and Evaluation of Experiences in 12 Developed Countries", *OECD Health Working Papers*, No. 54, OECD Publishing, Paris, http://dx.doi.org/10.1787/5kmbrcfms5g7-en.

Department of Health, Australia (2013), *Review of Australian Government Health Workforce Programs* (the Mason Review), May.

DREES – Direction de la recherche, des études, de l'évaluation et des statistiques (2014), *La démographie des médecins* [Medical Demography], Paris, April.

Health Workforce Australia (2012), *Health Workforce 2025 – Doctors, Nurses and Midwives – Vol. 1 and Vol. 2*, Adelaide, http://www.hwa.gov.au/sites/uploads/FinalReport_Volume1_FINAL-20120424.pdf.

Juraschek, S. et al. (2012), "United States Registered Nurse Workforce Report Card and Shortage Forecast", *Public Health Resources*, Paper No. 149, http://digitalcommons.unl.edu/publichealthresources/149.

Morgan, D. and R. Astolfi (2014), "Health Spending Continues to Stagnate in Many OECD Countries", *OECD Health Working Papers No. 68*, OECD Publishing, Paris, http://dx.doi.org/10.1787/5jz5sq5qnwf5-en.

OECD (2015), *Health at a Glance 2015: OECD Indicators,* OECD Publishing, Paris, http://dx.doi.org/10.1787/health_glance-2015-en.

OECD (2014a), *Health at a Glance: Europe 2014*, OECD Publishing, Paris, http://dx.doi.org/10.1787/health_glance_eur-2014-en.

OECD (2014b), *OECD Pensions Outlook 2014*, OECD Publishing, Paris, http://dx.doi.org/10.1787/9789264222687-en.

OECD (2008), *The Looming Crisis in the Health Workforce: How Can OECD Countries Respond?*, OECD Publishing, Paris, http://dx.doi.org/10.1787/9789264050440-en.

Pong, R.W. (2011), *Putting Up the Stethoscope for Good?*, CIHI, available at http://www.cihi.ca.

Seematter-Bagnoud, L. et al. (2007), *Offre et recours aux soins médicaux ambulatoires en Suisse*, Observatoire suisse de la santé.

Van der Windt, W. (2013), *Noticie Uitstroom medisch specialisten* [Note on the Exit of Medical Specialists], Kiwa Prismant, Amsterdam.

Chapter 3
Education and training for doctors and nurses: What's happening with *numerus clausus* policies?

By Liliane Moreira and Gaétan Lafortune (OECD Health Division)[1]

One of the most powerful policy levers governments can use to adjust the supply of doctors and nurses to projected demand is the so-called numerus clausus, *that is, the regulation of the number of students entering medical and nursing education programmes. This chapter describes the evolution of* numerus clausus *policies in OECD countries over the past 15 years and key challenges in achieving an adequate number and mix of different categories of health workers. Since 2000, most OECD countries have increased substantially the number of students admitted to medical and nursing education, in response to concerns about current or future staff shortages. This has often been accompanied by deliberate policies to increase more rapidly post-graduate training places in general medicine vis-à-vis other specialties to strengthen the primary care workforce. A number of OECD countries have also introduced or expanded training programmes for advanced practice nurses such as nurse practitioners also to increase access to primary care by relying more on non-physicians. Following a strong and steady expansion in training capacity, some countries now worry about a possible over-supply of graduates entering the labour market. How might governments use more wisely these* numerus clausus *policies and the large amount of public resources spent in training future health workers? This chapter stresses that the health workforce planning models that are guiding these policy decisions need to better factor changes in population health needs and in the scope of practice of different health care providers that might impact on their future demand. These models also need to take into account the growing international mobility of students and health workers, which makes it more complicated to determine the "right number" to train at a national level.*

This chapter has been produced with the financial assistance of the European Union. The views expressed herein can in no way be taken to reflect the official opinion of the European Union.

3.1. Introduction

Ensuring an adequate balance in the number and mix of health workers is essential for the proper functioning of health systems. An undersupply of physicians, for instance, can hamper access to health services for certain parts of the population, whereas an oversupply can lead to a loss of human capital and increase government cost pressures through supply-induced demand.

One key policy lever governments use to influence the supply of health workers is the regulation of admissions into education and training programmes, so-called *numerus clausus* (i.e. closed number) policies. Most OECD countries have used such policies for a few decades now, to regulate entry into health professionals' education programmes and post-graduate training in different specialties for doctors. This policy is usually implemented either by explicitly regulating the number of students admitted each year (i.e. quotas) and/or by limiting the public budget subsidising education and training places. Although this is clearly a powerful tool to adjust the supply of health workers, the effect of these policies are not felt immediately, as it takes a number of years to train new doctors, nurses and other health workers.

Ever since *numerus clausus* policies were introduced, both their legitimacy and management have been questioned. In several countries, *numerus clausus* policies have often been characterised by upward and downward phases, as a response to changing concerns about future shortages or surpluses of health care providers. This has sometime been called the "yo-yo" approach to fixing the *numerus clausus*. Determining the right number of student admissions has proven to be a challenge, given the wide range and uncertainty of factors affecting both the future demand and supply of health workers. In some countries, the discussions have focussed on improving the decision-making process by strengthening the information base and projection models supporting decisions around *numerus clausus* policies (Ono et al., 2013). One country at least, Australia, has recently taken the bold initiative of abandoning *numerus clausus* policies for most health-related university studies, with the exception of medical education, in an effort to open up entry into university education (see Box 3.2).

This chapter first describes the initial aim, rationale and historical evolution of *numerus clausus* policies in OECD countries, focussing on medical and nursing education given the preeminent role that doctors and nurses have traditionally played in OECD countries. Second, it reviews changes in *numerus clausus* policies in medical and nursing education since 2000 across a large number of OECD countries, considering whether there have been any changes in directions following the economic crisis in 2008. Third, it analyses trends in *numerus clausus* policies for medical post-graduate training programmes, contrasting admissions in general medicine with other medical specialties. Finally, it reviews the development of education and training programmes for nurses in advanced roles such as nurse practitioners (NPs), as an example of a "mid-level" professional role that might help reduce the need to train a greater number of doctors.

This chapter concludes that there is a need for a regular re-assessment of *numerus clausus* policies, taking into account changing economic circumstances and new innovations that may affect the future demand and supply of health workers. These regular re-assessments need to be based on robust health workforce planning models and data, which are broader in scope than the silo approach used so far. Greater considerations need to be given to the interactions among different health care providers and changing scopes of practice, as well as the growing internationalisation in health labour markets.

3.2. The evolution of *numerus clausus* policies in OECD countries, new challenges and need for regular adjustments

Since the 1970s, most OECD countries have regulated the number of students admitted in medical schools through *numerus clausus* policies. A number of reasons have steered most OECD countries to adopt these policies including: 1) recognition of the limited capacity in hospitals and other health care settings to provide practical training to new doctors, combined with an interest in selecting students deemed to be the most able to pursue long and complex medical studies; 2) interest in limiting the amount of public spending in medical education (given that these studies are costly and heavily subsidised in all countries); and 3) need to control the number of doctors entering the profession to avoid an oversupply of doctors and an increase in supply-induced demand. In addition, the length of medical studies itself (which can last around ten years to complete specialty training), justified planning and control over student intakes to avoid shortages or surpluses in the medium to longer term. While *numerus clausus* policies generally started in medical education, several countries extended their use to other education fields, including dentistry, pharmacy, midwifery and nursing.

Numerus clausus are usually implemented by fixing explicit quotas on admissions to medical and nursing education and post-graduate training programmes. Some countries such as Chile, Italy and the United States do not explicitly impose such quotas, but budgetary constraints at the national or sub-national level limit *de facto* the number of students admitted. Two countries – the Czech Republic and the Slovak Republic – report that they do not have a *numerus clausus* for medical education. However, the available data on admission or graduation rates suggest that the limited capacity in universities in these countries also impose constraints on the number of students admitted each year.

In France, *numerus clausus* policies for medical education were established in 1971, with explicit quotas taking effect in 1972. The explicit purpose of this measure was to match the number of medical students to hospitals' limited capacity to offer training places. Another less explicit reason was to curb the existing number of doctors and avoid adding undue pressures on expenditures in a system based on fee-for-services. Since 2009, *numerus clausus* policies in France also aim at addressing imbalances in the geographic distribution of doctors by using regional quotas, with limited success (ONDPS, 2015). As in several other countries, the setting of the *numerus clausus* in France has been characterised by large upward or downward fluctuation in admissions over time, reflecting changing concerns about either shortages or surpluses of doctors (see Box 3.1).[2]

In the Netherlands, *numerus clausus* in medical studies were initially introduced in 1976 to select only top students in a context where the number of applicants started to greatly exceed training capacities. Today, these quotas further aim at containing public costs related to the education and training programmes and restricting potential supply-induced demand (Ketel et al., 2012). The Ministry of Education, Culture and Science decides annually how many students will access medical education and various medical specialisations. Since 2000, this decision is based on recommendations from the Advisory Committee on Medical Manpower Planning (ACMMP), which has been tasked to regularly re-assess the projected demand and supply of doctors and other health professions (ACMMP, 2013).

Box 3.1. Changes in the *numerus clausus* for medical education in France

Following the decision to introduce a *numerus clausus* in France in 1971, the number of students admitted in medical education programmes started to decrease sharply a few years afterwards. It came down from nearly 9 000 students admitted per year in the mid-1970s to 3 500 in the 1990s, in response to concerns about a possible oversupply of doctors and the pressures that would put on health expenditures. From the end of the 1990s up to 2011, the numbers went back up to 8 000 students given growing concerns about foreseen shortages of doctors. Since then, between 2012 and 2014, the number of new students has been stable. Further decisions on *numerus clausus* are pending on new projections over future demand and supply of doctors. These new projections are expected to take into account several recent developments that will affect the future supply of doctors, including changing retirement patterns and growing numbers of foreign-trained physicians migrating to France.

Evolution of the *numerus clausus* for medical education in France, 1971-2013

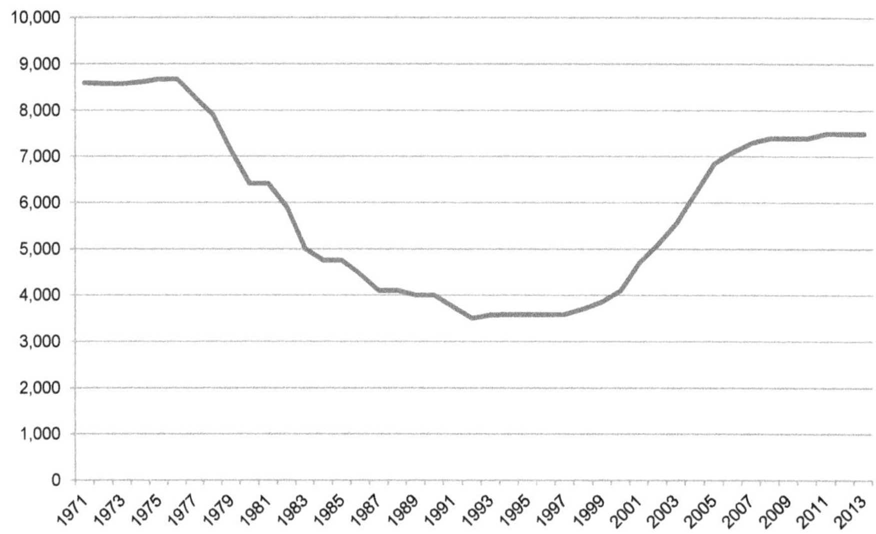

Source: ONDPS (2015), *Rapport 2013-2014: La régulation démographique des professionnels de santé par les flux d'étudiants, la situation démographique des chirurgiens-dentistes, bilan de la filiarisation*, Paris.

In Germany, the total number of places in medical education programmes available each year is decided at the state (*Länder*) level. From the total number of places available, 20% are allocated to high-school top performers, 20% for qualified applicants who have been on a waiting list for a certain period of time, and the remaining 60% are subject to admission criteria as defined by the universities (Miani et al., 2015). On average, the number of applicants tends to exceed by four times the number of places available (Chenot, 2009).

The majority of OECD countries also regulate student admissions in nursing education. However, its rationale is not as strong as for medical education, given that the duration and cost of training is lower for nursing, and there is less concern related to supply-induced demand.

Following a reform designed to open up entry into higher education, Australia recently abandoned its *numerus clausus* policies for most university education programmes, except for medical education. In 2008, the *Bradley Review of Higher Education* called for a shift from a supply-driven university admission system to a demand-driven one, allowing a greater number of young Australians to obtain a university degree (Bradley et al., 2008). Following the recommendations from this review, universities were given the freedom to determine how many students could be admitted in various fields. The Commonwealth Government assured funding would be available for every domestic student admitted to a public university. The only notable exception to this was the field of medicine, which continued to be regulated. A number of reasons led to the exclusion of medical education from this new demand-driven system in Australia, including the high cost of medical education and specialisation, and concerns that an oversupply of doctors would generate higher demand for health services and increase unnecessarily public costs for health care and prescription drugs. The recommendations from the Bradley review were also made following a rapid growth in the number of medical students, raising concerns over shortages of training places against the rising number of medical graduates (Kemp and Norton, 2014; see Box 3.2).

Box 3.2. Australia abandons *numerus clausus* policies for most university education programmes, except medicine

The following are excerpts from a 2014 report by Kemp and Norton. It summarises the rationale for keeping the *numerus clausus* policy for medical education in Australia, while entry into other university programmes was liberalised:

"In recommending the demand driven system, the Bradley report stated that the government could exclude a course if it wanted to control student or graduate numbers. Medicine is the only course specifically mentioned into the higher education funding legislation as outside the demand driven system. However, the legislation gives the minister power to exclude other courses (…) but no field of education other than medicine has so far been excluded from the demand driven system.

(…) The decision to exclude medicine was taken in consultation with the Health portfolio. Through the old system of allocated places there had already been rapid growth in medical student numbers in the years leading up to the demand driven system being announced. Following the establishment of several new medical schools the number of commencing medical students doubled between 2002 and 2009 to around 3 000.

Several reasons were given for capping medical student places. As in other health courses, rapid increases in student numbers had created a shortage of clinical training places for medical students. Medical training is very expensive, with Commonwealth contributions alone for a six year medical degree exceeding AUD 120 000. A further factor was a long-standing concern that too many doctors would result in additional unnecessary costs through Medicare and the Pharmaceutical Benefits Scheme." (Kemp and Norton, 2014).

In countries where *numerus clausus* policies exist, decisions on the number of students admitted each year are usually guided by projections about the future demand and supply of different categories of health workers. One complicating factor in making decisions on *numerus clausus* is the growing internationalisation of both university education and health labour markets, which are difficult to measure properly and forecast in health workforce planning models. This issue is particularly relevant in the European Union, where medical and nursing graduates who have obtained their degree in one country can easily get their degree recognised in another country, thereby reducing barriers to the mobility of students and workers.[3]

The growing number of doctors and nurses willing and able to move to other countries to seize better job opportunities raises important challenges for health workforce planning. This is the case not only for sending countries losing a sizable number of skilled workers they have trained, but also for destination countries, which could have trained fewer health workers to address any given demand. If destination countries do not consider inflows of foreign-trained doctors and nurses in determining their *numerus clausus*, this may lead to an over-supply of medical graduates. However, there is also a risk that countries which are net receivers of foreign-trained doctors or nurses may become complacent with this arrangement, and start free riding on the training efforts of other countries. Therefore, when deciding on *numerus clausus*, policy makers are confronted with a difficult balance between not overly relying on the training efforts of other countries to fulfil their own domestic needs, while recognising that both students and health workers will most likely be increasingly mobile in the future.

The Netherlands provides an interesting example of how the *numerus clausus* for medical education may need to be adjusted to reflect changes in the underlying data and assumptions around the mobility of doctors. In 2011, the quotas on admissions were increased following the expectation there would be fewer foreign-trained doctors coming into the Netherlands. Projections were suggesting that there would be substantial shortages of doctors across EU countries in the coming years. Three years later, the recommended quota was reduced as it was realised there had not been any reduction in the inflows of foreign-trained doctors. This example illustrates the growing complexity and uncertainty in setting a *numerus clausus* at a national level in a context where there are fewer barriers to the mobility of workers. It also highlights the need to regularly update these health workforce projections and to adapt *numerus clausus* decisions accordingly, as done in the Netherlands.

3.3. Trends in admissions in medical and nursing education

This section describes recent trends in admissions in medical and nursing education programmes in OECD countries. It starts by reviewing the general results from the *2012-13 OECD Health System Characteristics Survey*, which asked officials from Health Ministries to indicate whether there had been any changes in student intakes in medical and nursing education over the past five years (i.e., from 2007 to 2012). Table 3.1 summarises the responses to this question (further complemented by additional data sources, where needed).

Out of 31 OECD countries for which information is available, 21 increased the number of students admitted in medical education programmes between 2007 and 2012. For the remaining ten, the number remained relatively stable. With regards to nursing education, a vast majority of countries (21 out of 32) have also increased the number of students admitted between 2007 and 2012, while nine countries have maintained the number more or less constant during that same period. Only Portugal and the Slovak Republic have reduced the number of students admitted in nursing programmes. While the United Kingdom reported that the number of students admitted in nursing had been fairly constant in the United Kingdom as a whole, the number decreased in England.

Most countries reported to have increased student admissions for both medical and nursing programmes from 2007 and 2012, but there are some exceptions. In Italy and Poland, the intake of medical students increased, whereas the intake of nursing students remained constant. In Finland, Korea and Mexico, the opposite was reported, with an increase in nursing education intake, whereas admissions to medical education remained more or less stable.

The following sub-sections analyse in more detail trends in admissions in medical and nursing education over a longer time period for a subset of OECD countries. Annex 3.A2 provides additional data on the number of graduates from medical and nursing education programmes since 2005, for nearly all OECD countries, based on responses to the annual OECD/Eurostat/WHO-Europe Joint Questionnaire.

Table 3.1. Changes to medical and nursing education intake, OECD countries, 2007 to 2012

	Medical education intake	Nursing education intake
Australia	Increase	Increase
Austria	Constant	[No reply]
Belgium	Increase	Increase
Canada	Increase	Increase
Chile	Increase	Increase
Czech Republic	Constant	Constant
Denmark	Increase	Increase
Estonia	[No reply]	Increase
Finland	Constant	Increase
France	Constant	Constant
Germany	Increase	Increase
Greece	Constant	Constant
Hungary	Constant	Constant
Iceland	Constant	Constant
Ireland	Increase	Increase
Israel	Increase	Increase
Italy	Increase	Constant
Japan	Increase	Increase
Korea	Constant	Increase
Luxembourg	Non applicable (no medical schools)	Constant
Mexico	Constant	Increase
Netherlands	Increase*	Increase
New Zealand	Increase	Increase
Norway	Increase	Increase
Poland	Increase	Constant (with year-to-year fluctuations)
Portugal	Increase	Decrease
Slovak Republic	Increase	Decrease
Slovenia	Increase	Increase
Spain	Increase	Increase
Sweden	Increase	Increase
Switzerland	Increase	Increase
Turkey	[No reply]	[No reply]
United Kingdom	Constant	Constant (with variations in different parts)
United States	Increase	Increase

* In the Netherlands, student intakes in medical education increased in 2011 and 2012 following recommendations from the 2010 report from the ACMMP, based on the assumption that the number of foreign-trained doctors coming in the Netherlands would decrease. However, this reduction did not occur, so the follow-up report in 2013 recommended a reduction of the admission numbers back to its 2010 level.

Source: OECD Health System Characteristics Survey 2012, complemented with other national sources (see Annex 3.A3).

Trends in medical education admissions since 2000

Figure 3.1 shows trends in medical education admission numbers since 2000 in 18 OECD countries. In most of these countries, the number of students admitted in medical education has increased markedly since 2000 (though at different paces). In Finland, France, the Netherlands and the United Kingdom, most of the increase occurred in the early 2000s with the number stabilising afterwards, whereas in Australia, Canada, New Zealand, Portugal and Sweden the increase continued steadily throughout the period.

Figure 3.1. Student intake in medical education, selected OECD countries, 2000-13 (or nearest years)

Index (Baseline year = 100)

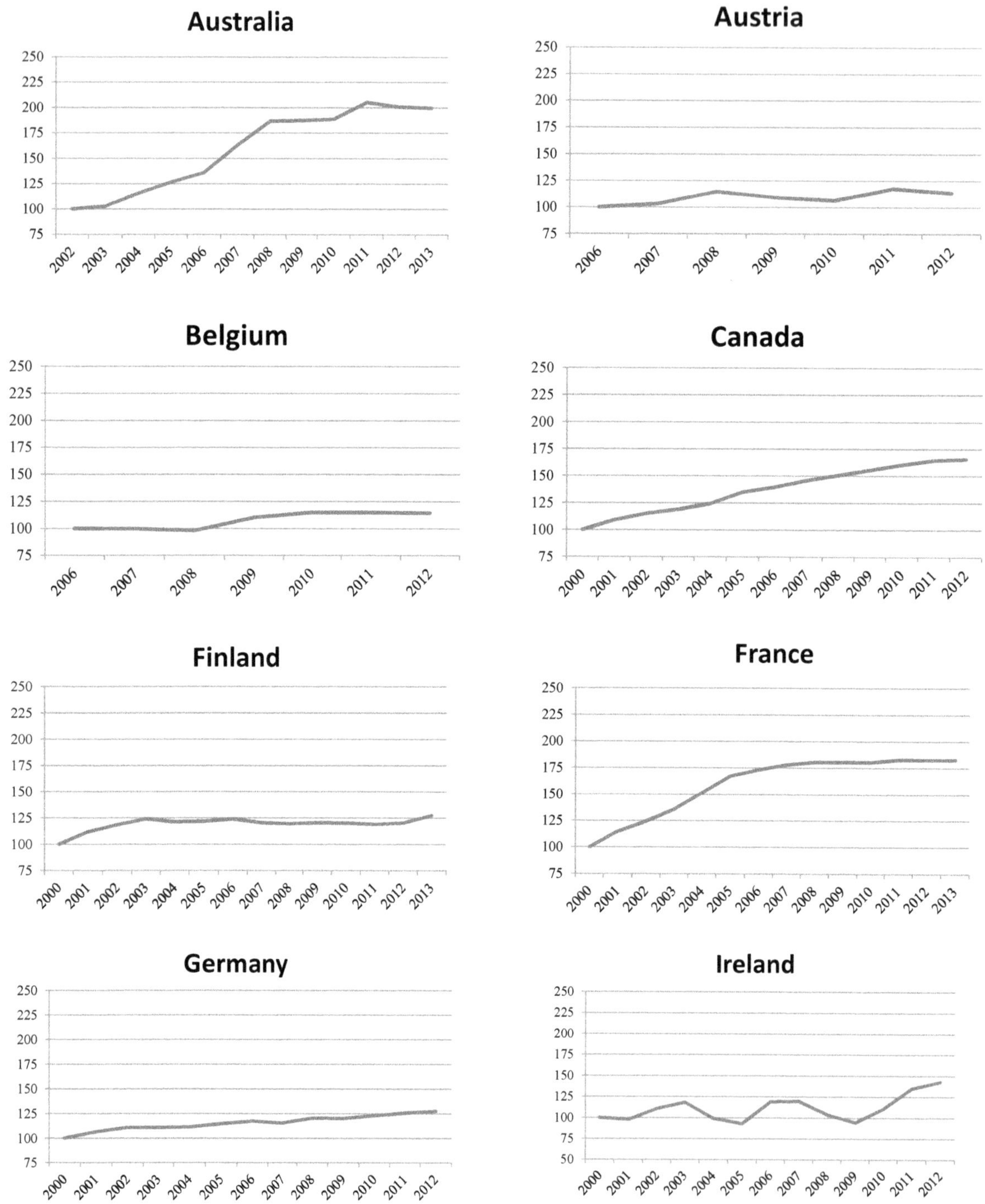

Figure 3.1. Student intake in medical education, selected OECD countries, 2000-13 (or nearest years) *(cont.)*

Index (Baseline year = 100)

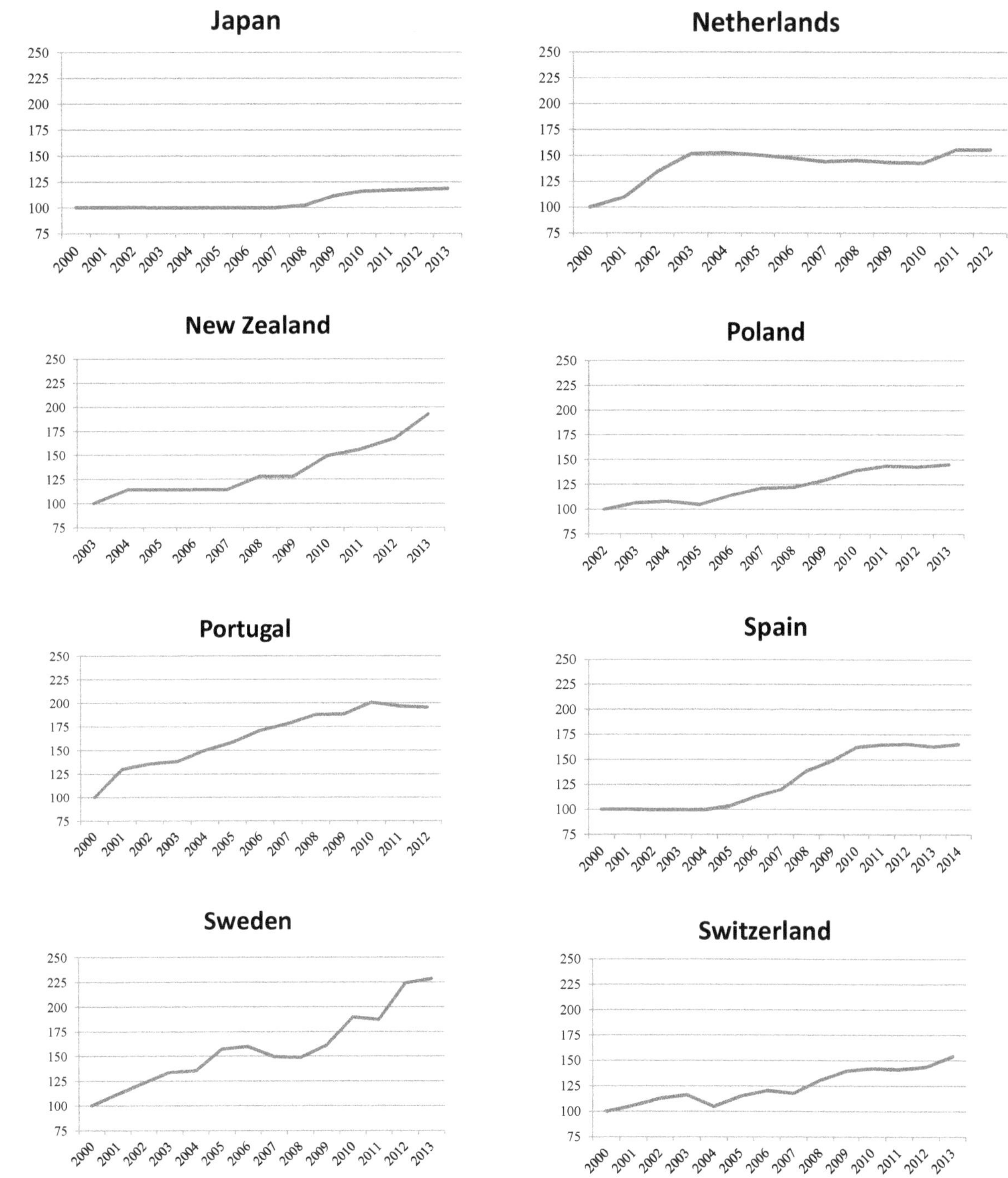

Figure 3.1. Student intake in medical education, selected OECD countries, 2000-13 (or nearest years) *(cont.)*

Index (Baseline year = 100)

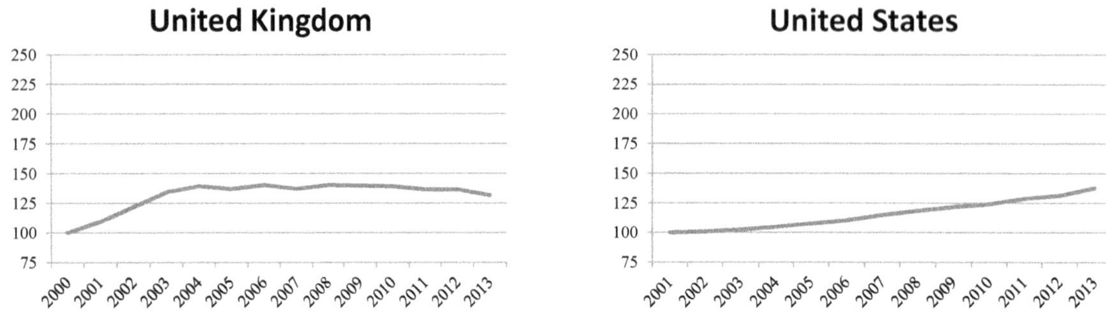

Note: For both Japan and France, the annual quotas (*numerus clausus*) set by governments are used as a proxy for actual student intakes. However, in France, there has been a gradual increase in the number of additional places for medical students beyond what is set in the main *numerus clausus*, with the number of such additional places rising from 42 places in 2001 (representing 0.9% of the main *numerus clausus*) to 536 in 2013 (representing 7.2% of the main *numerus clausus*) (ONDPS, 2015).

Source: Please refer to Annex 3.A3, Table 3.A3.1.

StatLink http://dx.doi.org/10.1787/888933326116

In Australia, admissions to medical education doubled between 2002 and 2013, with most of the growth occurring between 2002 and 2008. This large expansion was made possible by an increase in the number of medical programmes offered (seven new medical programmes have received accreditation since 2000) and fuelled by a rise in the number of both domestic and international students (see Box 3.3). The increase in the number of international medical students was prompted by a government decision to support their stay in Australia upon graduation and allow their medical registration (Joyce et al., 2007; Health Workforce Australia, 2012). However, this strong rise in both domestic and international students has created pressures on the availability of post-graduate training places. Most, but not all, international and domestic graduates have been able to find post-graduate training places (Hawthorne, 2012).

Box 3.3. The growing internationalisation of medical and nursing education

The internationalisation of medical and nursing education is a growing phenomenon in OECD countries. Growing numbers of students are pursuing medical education in a foreign country, often because they were not admitted in their country of origin. This demand from students is supported by a growing number of medical schools which are interested in offering places to foreign students.

In Australia, for instance, the number of international students enrolled in medical and nursing schools has increased strongly since 2002 (see table below), with many universities viewing international students as a way to maintain or expand their capacity and bring in more revenues by paying full tuition fees (Hawthorne, 2012).

International Student Enrolments in Medicine and Nursing, Australia, 2002 to 2013

	2002	2003	2004	2005	2006	2007	2008	2009	2010	2011	2012	2013
Medicine	367	378	421	460	426	436	499	487	529	529	651	636
Nursing	397	604	902	1 285	1 708	2 346	2 487	2 710	2 799	2 558	2 384	2 579

Source: Medical Deans (2014) and Higher Education Statistics (2014).

In Canada, there has also been a strong growth in the number of students admitted in medical schools, with the number increasing by two-thirds between 2000 and 2012. Each province determines how many students will be admitted in their medical schools, based on their projections of physician requirements and their education and financial capacity.

The United States has also experienced a substantial increase in the number of students admitted in medical schools, albeit at a slower rate than in Australia and Canada. Between 2001 and 2013, student intakes grew by over 33% with most of the rise occurring after 2005. In 2006, following projections that there would be a growing shortage of doctors, the Association of American Medical Colleges (AAMC) proposed a 30% increase in student enrolment over the following decade (AAMC, 2006). Two main factors have supported the increase in student intakes in the United States: 1) after two decades of stagnation, the number of medical schools increased from 124 in 2005 to 145 in 2013;[4] and 2) existing medical schools have expanded the number of students by more than 10% on average from 2002 to 2012 (AAMC, 2012). The number of Americans studying medicine abroad has also increased, notably in Caribbean countries, but generally with the intention of coming back to the United States to complete their post-graduate training. However, the number of residency posts is not keeping pace with the growing number of domestic or foreign-trained graduates wishing to complete their medical training, which is leading to a bottleneck (Iglehart, 2013). Unless the number of residency posts increases substantially in the coming years, it will become increasingly difficult for medical graduates from a foreign university to find a residency and ultimately practice in the United States.

In the Netherlands, student intake in medical education increased by 50% between 2000 and 2003. From 2003 to 2010, the number remained relatively stable or even declined slightly, until it went up again in 2011 and 2012. This last rise has been driven by concerns over an expected decrease in the number of foreign-trained doctors coming into the Netherlands following expected shortages of doctors in Europe (ACMMP, 2010). However, as previously noted, these concerns did not materialise. Hence, the 2013 ACMMP report recommended reducing the admission numbers back to their 2010 level (ACMMP, 2013).

In the United Kingdom, admissions in medical education increased rapidly between 2000 and 2004, stabilising after that. In 2013, the number of students admitted in medical schools decreased slightly for the first time. This followed a recommendation from the Health and Education National Strategic Exchange to reduce by 2% medical school intakes in 2013 based on a projected oversupply of doctors (Department of Health, 2012).

In France, there has been a large increase in the *numerus clausus* since 2000, with most of the growth occurring between 2000 and 2006. The annual quotas for entry in medical education increased from 4 100 in 2000 to 7 100 in 2006. As noted in Box 3.1, this sharp increase started in the late 1990s following a period when *numerus clausus* was reduced (from over 8 000 students per year up to the mid-1970s to less than 4 000 per year throughout the 1990s). In recent years, the *numerus clausus* in France has remained unchanged, given the lack of robust and up-to-date projections regarding the future supply and demand for doctors. The most recent projections are based on 2007 data as the baseline year, and the hypotheses underlying the main scenario have proven to under-estimate the number of incoming foreign-trained doctors and the retention rate of doctors beyond the "standard" retirement age, leading to an underestimation of the supply of doctors in 2015 (ONDPS, 2015).

In Portugal, admissions to medical education doubled between 2000 and 2010 (rising from approximately 800 in 2000 to 1 600 in 2010). As in other countries, this followed concerns over future physician shortages. However, a recent projection exercise indicated that there may be an oversupply of around 4 000 to 9 000 medical specialists in Portugal by 2025 under some assumptions, including a retirement age of 70 (Santana et al., 2014).

Figure 3.2 examines the impact of the recent economic crisis on *numerus clausus* policies for medical education in OECD countries. Overall, the economic crisis does not seem to have had any major influence on *numerus clausus* policies, with countries continuing to focus on the medium- to longer-term outlook rather than reacting to the short-term cyclical downturn. In Portugal, Australia, Germany, Canada and Spain, after strong growth prior to 2008, admission growth rates slowed down. In Japan, Switzerland, Poland, New Zealand and Sweden, the intake of medical students grew more rapidly after 2008, reflecting policy decisions to increase the supply of domestically-trained doctors in addressing projected shortages. In the United Kingdom, as noted above, most of the growth in medical student admissions occurred between 2000 and 2004, and there was a small reduction in 2013.

Figure 3.2. Average annual growth rates in admissions to medical education, selected OECD countries, pre- and post-crisis

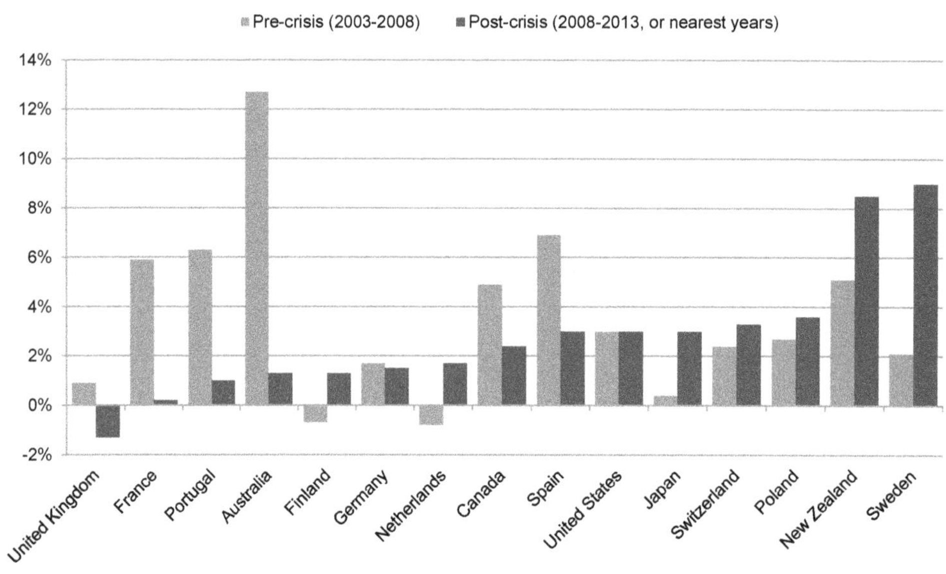

Note: Countries are ranked from the lowest to the highest average annual growth rate in admissions, post-crisis.

Source: Please refer to Annex 3.A3, Table 3.A3.1.

StatLink http://dx.doi.org/10.1787/888933326121

Trends in nursing education admissions since 2000

In the ten OECD countries for which data have been collected, student admissions in nursing education have also expanded substantially since 2000, with the exception of Portugal and the United Kingdom (England) where the numbers have come down since the mid-2000s (Figure 3.3). In Australia and the United States, admissions growth has been fairly steady throughout the period, reflecting concerns about current or future shortages of nurses.

Figure 3.3. Student intake in nursing education, selected OECD countries, 2000-13 (or nearest years)

(Index: Baseline year = 100)

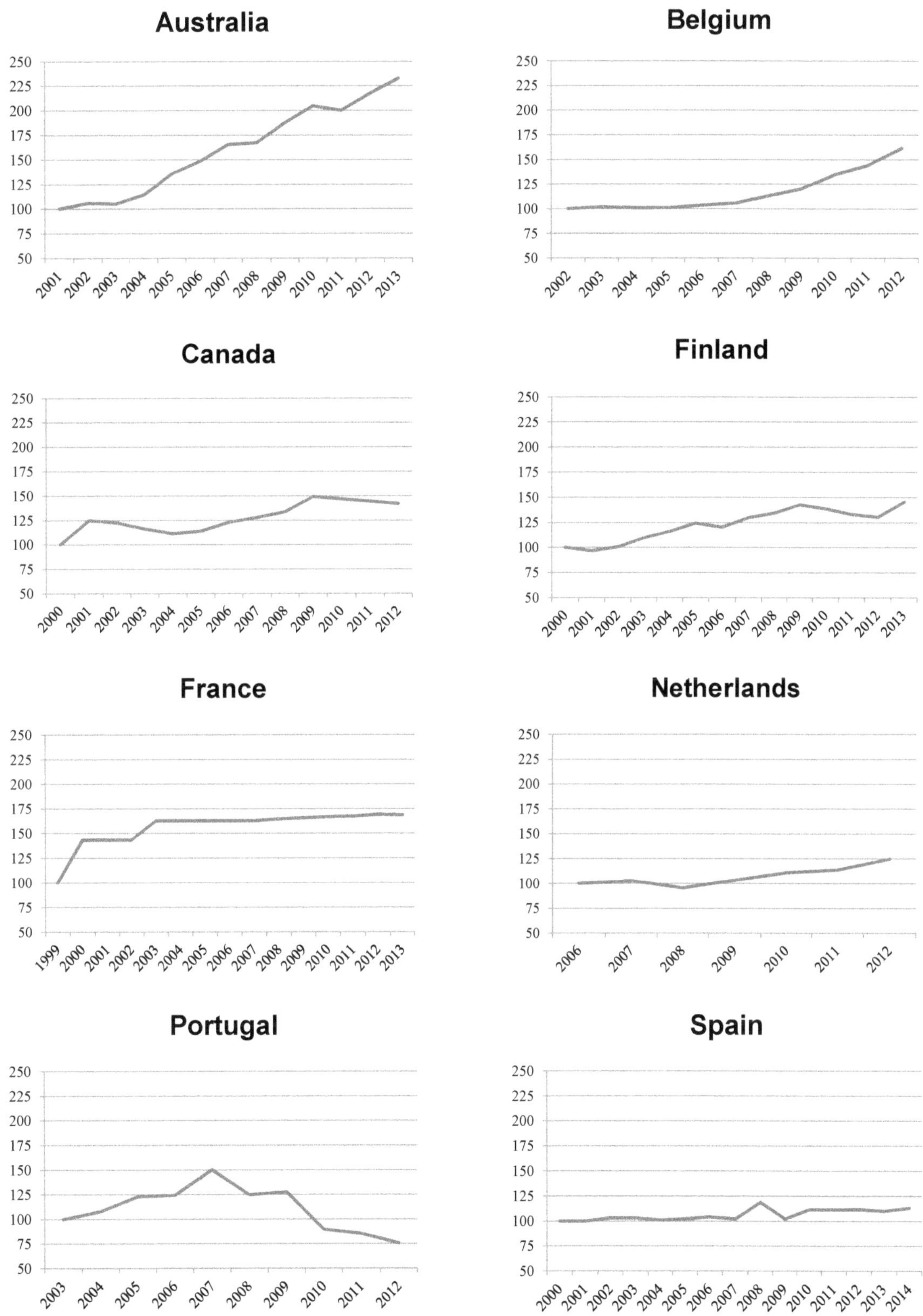

Figure 3.3. Student intake in nursing education, selected OECD countries, 2000-13 (or nearest years) *(cont.)*

(Index: Baseline year = 100)

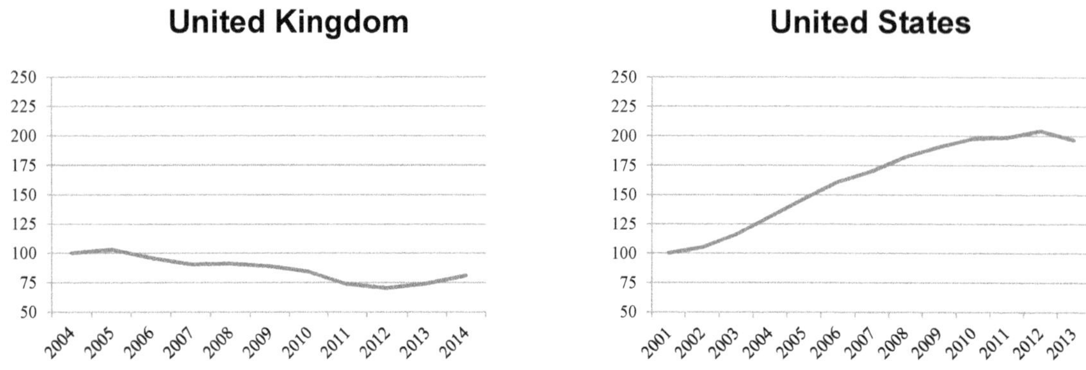

Note: For the United States, the number of graduates is used as a proxy for the number of students admitted to nursing education. For France, the annual quotas (*numerus clausus*) established by the government are used as a proxy for the number of students admitted to nursing education. For Spain, the nursing education programme was changed from a medium level to a higher-level diploma in 2008: many nurses were admitted during that year to complete their diploma, explaining the peak. For the United Kingdom, the data relate to training places for adult nurses in England only.

Source: Please refer to Annex 3.A3, Table 3.A3.2.

StatLink http://dx.doi.org/10.1787/888933326131

In Australia, the number of students admitted to nursing schools more than doubled between 2001 and 2013, rising from 8 122 to 18 885. This expansion was supported by a freeze in tuition fees for students in nursing at their 2004 level, a reduction in debt repayments for graduates going on to work as nurses, and an increase in the number of foreign students (Health Workforce Australia, 2013). In addition, following the Bradley review of 2008, *numerus clausus* policies for entry in nursing education were abandoned (Box 3.2). Some universities lowered entrance requirements to attract more students, and the capacity of certain universities was stretched. Since the introduction of this liberal system, admissions in nursing programmes have increased by 25% between 2009 and 2013, with most of this growth driven by an increase in the number of Australian students (the number of foreign students remained relatively stable). However, the growth rate following this reform was not greater than the growth rate when the government was still exercising greater control on entry. In fact, during the four years that preceded the reform, the growth rate in the number of students admitted in nursing programmes in Australia was even greater, reaching almost 40%. This illustrates how a regulated system (based on a *numerus clausus* policy) can lead to a similar increase in the number of students as a liberal one, with the main difference being who is making the decision and on what basis. Following these steady increases in the number of students admitted in nursing programmes under both the regulated and unregulated systems, one emerging issue in Australia is that there may no longer be enough entry positions to absorb all the new graduates in the labour market. A significant proportion of new domestic nursing graduates in recent years have been unable to secure suitable employment in at least certain areas of the country (Health Workforce Australia, 2014).

In the United States, the number of graduates from registered nurses (RN) programmes nearly doubled between 2001 and 2013, rising from 102 009 to 200 341 (according to data from the National League for Nursing). Following a marked decrease in student intakes during the 1990s, a 2004 report from the Department of Health and Human Services projected that there would be a significant shortage of RNs by 2020 if no change was made (Health and Human Services, 2004). The rapid expansion in admissions in nursing education programmes over the past decade was driven by successful campaigns to promote the profession and by a strong increase in the number of RN programmes. However, as in Australia, there are now concerns that graduates from nursing education programmes may soon exceed demand. The most recent projections estimate that, if student admission rates remain at their 2013 level, there will be an over-supply of more than 300 000 RNs by 2025. An over-supply is also expected for Licensed Practice Nurses (Health and Human Services, 2014).

In France, *numerus clausus* policies for entry in nursing education programmes have also increased substantially since 1999. The number of places grew by nearly 70% (rising from around 18 400 places in 1999 to over 31 000 in 2013). However, most of this growth occurred in the academic year of 2000/01 when the annual quota was increased by 43% (by 8 000 places). This sharp increase was driven by a projected reduction in the supply of nurses resulting from the reduction of working time to 35 hours per week, as well as the expectation that a large number of nurses would retire in the following years.

In Belgium, the number of students admitted in nursing has increased strongly since 2008. However, this growth has been driven to a large extent by foreign students who, in most cases, do not stay in Belgium once they have completed their studies.

By contrast, in the United Kingdom (England), the number of training places for adult nurses came down by about 25% between 2004 and 2012, before starting to rise again since 2013 in response to concerns about substantial shortages.

In Portugal, following an increase in intakes up to 2007, the number of students entering in nursing schools has been reduced by half between 2007 and 2012. Nurses were not spared from the austerity measures following the financial and economic crisis, which included cuts in nurses' salaries, a freeze of promotions and reductions in hiring. In 2012, graduates from nursing programmes were facing major difficulties in finding jobs, with many turning to temporary employment agencies (European Federation of Nurses Associations, 2012).

Figure 3.4 examines to what extent the recent economic crisis might have had an impact on admissions to nursing education in different countries. In Australia, Finland, Canada and the United States, admission rates continued to grow after the economic crisis but at a slower rate than during the pre-crisis years. In Ireland and Belgium, the number of students admitted has grown even faster since 2008, although as already noted the growth in Belgium was driven to a large extent by an increase in foreign students in Belgian nursing schools. By contrast, in Portugal admissions in nursing have significantly come down following the economic crisis.

Figure 3.4. Average annual growth rates in admissions to nursing education, selected OECD countries, pre- and post-crisis

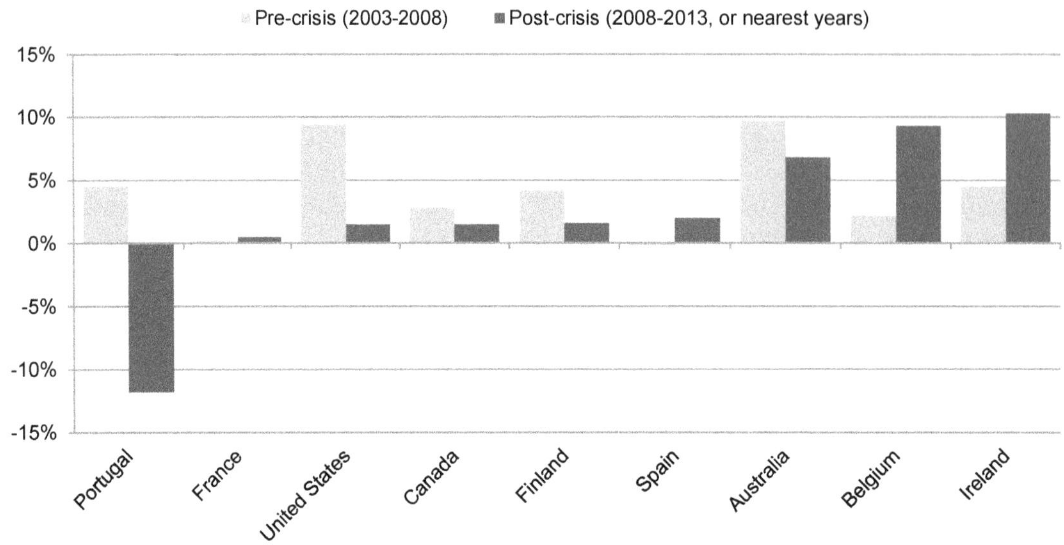

Note: Countries are ranked from the lowest to the highest average annual growth rate in admissions, post-crisis. For Spain, the periods considered are 2003-09 (pre-crisis) and 2009-14 (post-crisis).

Source: Please refer to Annex 3.A3, Table 3.A3.2.

StatLink http://dx.doi.org/10.1787/888933326148

3.4. Post-graduate training for doctors: The quest for a better balance between general practitioners and other medical specialists

As is the case for initial medical education, many OECD countries also regulate the number of places and/or financial resources allocated for post-graduate medical training. In recent years, beyond increasing the overall numbers of students in medical schools, several OECD countries have also taken steps to adjust the mix of specialty training places to modify the composition of the medical workforce. To increase the supply of general practitioners (GPs) and strengthen primary care, several countries opened up a greater number of places in general medicine.[5]

A number of factors influence the choice of specialty training of medical graduates beyond the number of places available. These include the length of the training period, the employment and remuneration prospects, and other aspects related to the working conditions (Creed et al., 2010; Mirvis, 2013). To be effective, a policy aiming to stir medical graduates towards general practice needs to address these factors in a coherent way.

In Canada, the number of first-year post-graduate training places in family medicine (i.e., general practice) more than doubled between 2000 and 2013, rising from around 600 to over 1 350, as part of a national effort to strengthen access to family doctors and primary care for the whole population (Figure 3.5). The number of training places in family medicine increased steadily during that period, at a rate of about 10% per year. Because this was accompanied by an almost equally strong rise in the number of places in other medical and surgical specialties, the share of all post-graduate training places in family medicine only increased moderately from 39% in 2000 to 44% in 2013.

Training in family medicine in Canada lasts a minimum of two years compared with three to five years for other medical or surgical specialties, though a growing number of trainees in general medicine are now doing an optional third year for sub-specialisation. In most cases, this additional year of training is taken in emergency family medicine, with very few trainees opting so far for sub-specialising in care for the elderly (Pong, 2012).[6]

As is the case in several other countries, in Canada, more women than men choose their post-graduate training in family medicine (CAPER, 2014). Given that women represent a growing share of students in initial medical education, this should help increase further the number of applicants to fill family medicine posts.

Figure 3.5. Places filled in medical post-graduate training, Canada, 2000-13

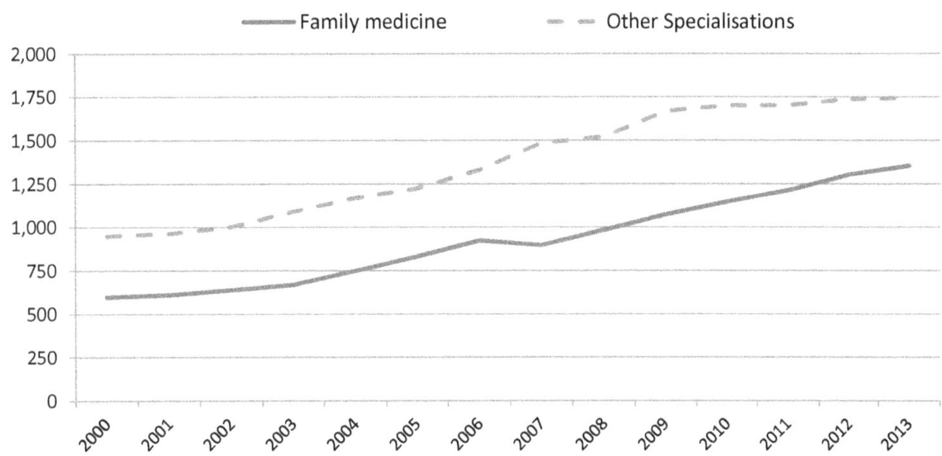

Source: Canadian Post-M.D Education Registry (2015), Data Tables (accessed 15 January 2015).

StatLink http://dx.doi.org/10.1787/888933326153

In the United States, the number of trainees in family medicine and internal medicine remained relatively stable between 2000 and 2012, but started to increase in 2013 and went up again in 2014. As a result, from 2012 to 2014, the number of training places in family medicine grew by 15% and in internal medicine by 23%.[7] The number of trainees also grew significantly in other medical or surgical specialisations, therefore the share of trainees in family medicine and internal medicine only increased slightly (Figure 3.6).

The recent increase in the number of training places in family medicine and internal medicine was driven by concerns about future shortages of generalists. Not only is a large number of generalists expected to retire over the next ten years, but there is also a projected growth in the demand for their services linked to an ageing population and expansion of insurance coverage (Petterson et al., 2012). A 2013 report from the Department of Health and Human Services projected that there may be a shortage of about 20 000 primary care doctors in 2020, based on the 2010 graduation rates (HHS, 2013). Some additional measures may be required to increase further the training of family doctors and other primary care doctors. One option includes increasing teaching hospitals resources so that more students are offered training in family medicine and other primary care specialisations. Another option is to increase the use of nurse practitioners (NPs) and physician assistants (PAs) to reduce the projected shortage of primary care doctors in the United States.

Figure 3.6. Places filled in medical post-graduate training, United States, 2000-14

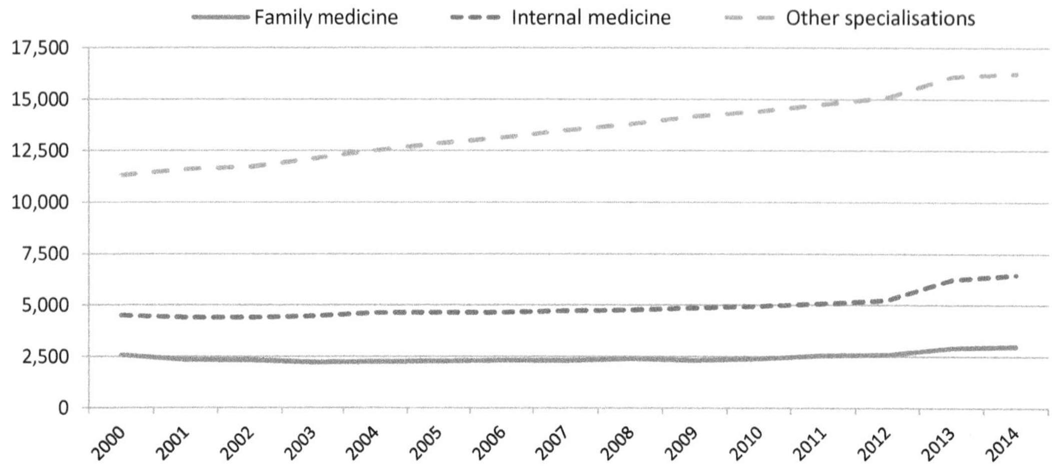

Source: National Resident Matching Program, Results and Data Reports (2004, 2008, 2014).

StatLink http://dx.doi.org/10.1787/888933326165

In France, over the past ten years important efforts have been made to increase the number of post-graduate training places in general medicine (Figure 3.7). Since 2004, the number of training places available in general medicine has increased more rapidly than in other specialisations. However, these places have not always been filled. In fact, until 2011, there was a fairly large gap between the positions available and those actually filled. This gap can be explained by a number of factors including the limited capacity of teaching hospitals and other trainers to provide internship positions in general medicine and the unwillingness of new medical graduates to choose general medicine. This gap was closed down in 2012 and 2013 as the number of places available was slightly reduced and the number of places filled increased.

Figure 3.7. Places filled in medical post-graduate training, France, 2004-13

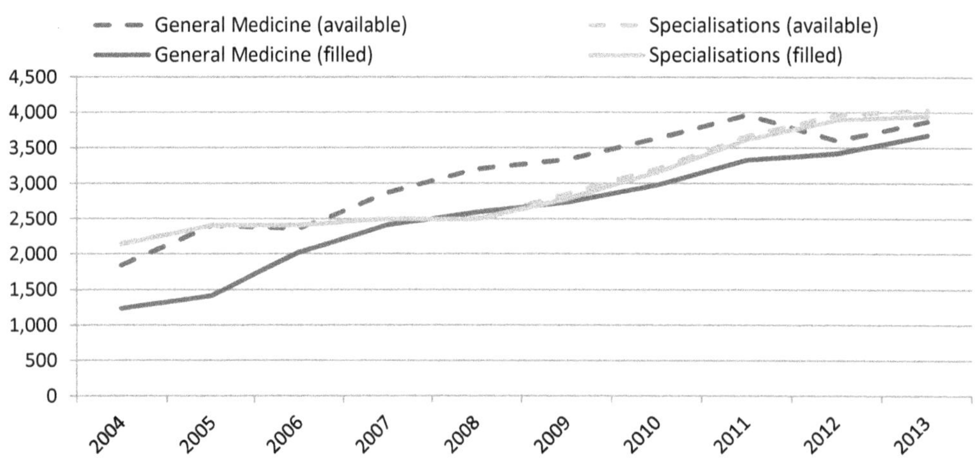

Source: DREES (2011), "Les affectations des étudiants en médecine à l'issue des épreuves classantes nationales en 2010", Études et Résultats, No. 767 ; DREES (2014), "Les affectations des étudiants en médecine à l'issue des épreuves classantes nationales en 2013", *Études et Résultats*, No. 894, Paris.

StatLink http://dx.doi.org/10.1787/888933326178

In the Netherlands, the number of post-graduate training places filled in general medicine was fairly stable up to 2008, when it started to rise slowly (Figure 3.8). Between 2008 and 2012, the number of these post-graduate training places filled increased from 537 to 638, an increase of almost 20%. Yet, this growth was more modest than the number of places filled in other medical and surgical specialties which grew by 30%. In 2013, the ACMMP recommended that the number of places in general medicine training remain the same as in 2012, while the number of places in other specialisations should reduce back to their level of 2009 and 2010, given concerns about a possible over-supply of doctors in certain specialties. As previously noted, these concerns were partly linked to previous projections of a possible reduction in inflow of foreign-trained medical specialists in the Netherlands (ACMMP, 2013). In assessing the future demand for GPs, the ACMMP also took into account the fact that a growing number of PAs and NPs could respond to the demand for primary care services. This more comprehensive approach of looking at the primary health care workforce as a whole is quite innovative as interactions and possible substitutions between different health care providers are often neglected in health workforce planning models and policy discussions in other countries.

Figure 3.8. Places filled in medical post-graduate training, the Netherlands, 2002-12

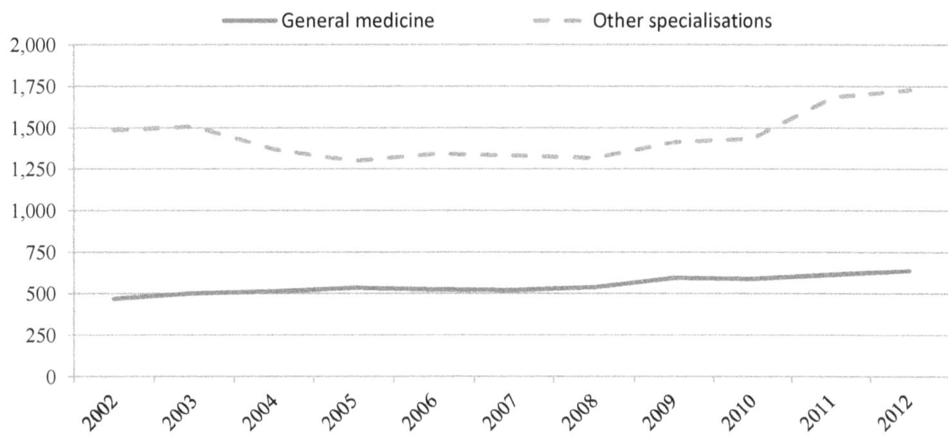

Source: ACMMP – Advisory Committee on Medical Manpower Planning (2013), *The 2013 Recommendations for Medical Specialist Training*, Capaciteitsorgaan, Utrecht.

StatLink http://dx.doi.org/10.1787/888933326185

In Spain, the number of post-graduate places filled in general medicine remained fairly stable between 2000 and 2010 while the number of places in other medical and surgical specialisations increased steadily (Figure 3.9). The number of places filled in other medical and surgical specialisations grew from around 3 300 in 2000 to 5 000 in 2010, a rise of approximately 50%. As a result, the proportion of trainees in general medicine fell from 36% in 2000 to 28% in 2010. Since 2010, the number of internship places in both general medicine and other specialties has started to decrease. In 2012, the Spanish Ministry of Health called for a reduction in the number of places available in medical schools, following the results from new health workforce planning exercises projecting surpluses and the lack of capacity of the health system to absorb all new graduates.

Figure 3.9. Places filled in medical post-graduate training, Spain, 2000-13

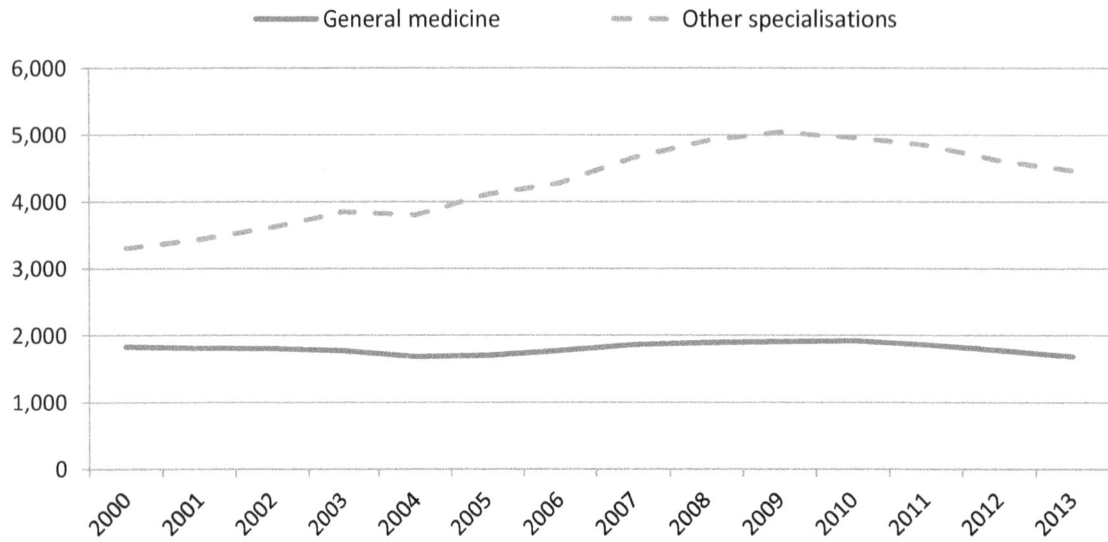

Source: Ministerio de Sanidad, Servicios Sociales e Igualdad [Ministry of Health, Social Services and Equality], 2015.

StatLink http://dx.doi.org/10.1787/888933326190

In a 2011 survey, Spanish medical graduates were invited to indicate which factors were most relevant for choosing their specialty area. Employment prospects came out as the most important reason. This probably explains the growing number and share of medical graduates applying for general medicine training in recent years, reflecting the perception that there may be greater employment opportunities in this field (Harris et al., 2013). However, since the offer of training places in general medicine has started to come down in recent years, one can infer that a lower percentage of applicants are actually getting a place.

Figure 3.10 shows the mix of students admitted in post-graduate training in general medicine vis-à-vis other medical specialties in six OECD countries in 2013 (or the nearest year). In France, the ratio of students in general medicine reaches nearly 50%, reflecting a deliberate effort to reach an almost equal balance. In Canada and the United Kingdom (England), the proportion of students pursuing general medicine training is also relatively high (over 40%). In England, the government mandated Health Education England in 2013 to reach 50% of medical graduates in GP training by 2015. This would mean that around 3 250 students would pursue this specialisation on an annual basis, up from the around 2 700 in recent years. A GP taskforce was created to come up with a set of recommendations on how to achieve this goal (NHS, 2014).

Figure 3.10. Share of students admitted in general medicine and other specialisations, selected OECD countries, 2013 (or nearest year)

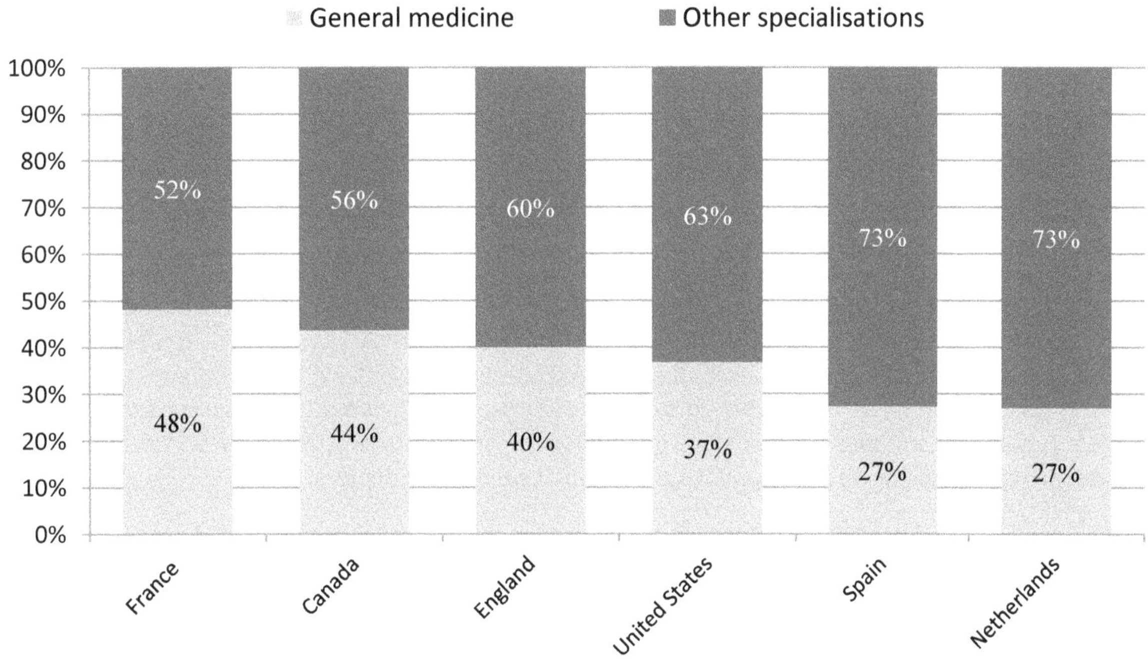

Note: In the United States, general medicine includes students admitted to both family medicine and internal medicine.

Source: See sources in Figures 3.5 to 3.9.

StatLink http://dx.doi.org/10.1787/888933326201

3.5. Advanced education for nurses: The development of programmes for nurse practitioners

Many OECD countries are seeking to re-organise health service delivery to better respond to changing population health care needs by reviewing the roles of different health professionals, including those of nurses. Developing new and more advanced roles for nurses beyond the traditional scope of their practice is considered in many countries as a promising approach to improve access to care while helping to contain cost (Delamaire and Lafortune, 2010). This expansion is based on the prospect that advanced practice nurses (APNs) may play an increasing role in service delivery in primary care or in hospital. In primary care, advance practice nurses may take new tasks such as being the first point of contact for patients with minor problems, prescribing pharmaceuticals or tests, and routinely monitoring patients with chronic conditions.

The first education programmes in advanced nursing to train nurse practitioners (NPs) were created in the United States in the 1960s, when the University of Colorado pioneered a new NP certificate programme. Since then, these programmes have spread throughout the United States, as well as in Canada, the United Kingdom and several other countries. In most countries where positions for NPs now exist, the educational requirement to obtain these positions is generally a master's degree although there are some exceptions (for example, a university bachelor's degree is still sufficient in certain parts of Canada).[8]

In the United States more than 100 000 NPs were working in the health system in 2010, totalling about 5.5% of all RNs, with half of them working in primary care (HRSA, 2013). The number of NPs is expected to continue to grow in the coming years, given increases in admissions and graduation rates, and further growth in the demand for their services. Between 2001 and 2012, the number of graduates from NP programmes in the United States more than doubled, rising from around 7 000 in 2001 to over 14 000 in 2012 (Figure 3.11). This number increased further to 15 000 in 2013 (AANP, 2015).

For the past 20 years, a master's degree is required to become a NP (or any other recognised advanced practice nurse) in the United States. In 2013, 95% of NPs had at least a master's degree, up from 62% in 2000 (AANP, 2013). In 2004, the American Association of Colleges of Nurses and the National Council of State Boards of Nursing proposed that the minimum requirement for advanced nursing practice be raised further to a "doctor of nursing practice" (DNP) to be imposed from 2015 onwards. While this change would not have any consequence on current NPs and other APNs with a master's degree (who would still be able to continue to practice), it would add more years of education and training for the new generation of advanced practice nurses, therefore narrowing the gap with the education and training of medical doctors.

Figure 3.11. Graduates from nurse practitioner programmes, United States, 2001-12

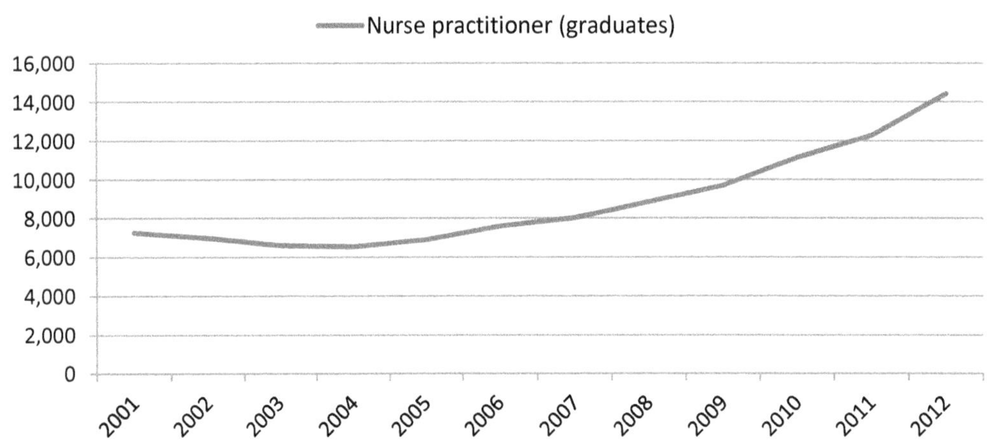

Source: Health Resources and Services Administration, Bureau of Health (2013).

StatLink http://dx.doi.org/10.1787/888933326218

An increased supply of NPs is seen as an important response to the growing demand for health services related to ageing population and the expansion in health insurance coverage under the Affordable Care Act. However, there are now some concerns that the growing number of NP graduates might lead to an over-supply in the coming years. Based on a 2013 health workforce projection carried out by the Department of Health and Human Services, the projected growth in the demand for NPs between 2010 and 2020 may fall short of the projected growth in their supply, leading to the potential unemployment or under-employment of new graduates from these programmes. Such an over-supply might be even greater for PAs working in primary care (Table 3.2). However, under a scenario whereby NPs would provide a greater share of services in primary care, the demand for their services would be higher and the potential over-supply smaller (Health Resources and Services Administration, 2013).

Table 3.2. Projected supply and demand for primary care nurse practitioners and physician assistants, United States, 2010 and 2020

Provider type/specialty	2010	2020
Supply		
Nurse practitioners	55 400	72 100
Physician assistants	27 700	43 900
Demand		
Nurse practitioners	55 400	64 700
Physician assistants	27 700	32 700
Supply and demand		
Nurse practitioners	*	7 400
Physician assistants	*	11 200

Note: No data was available for estimating if there were shortages of NPs and PAs in the baseline year (2010).

Source: Health Resources and Services Administration (2013).

In Canada, the first NPs appeared more or less at the same time as in the United States in the mid-1960s, mainly to respond to shortages of doctors in rural and remote regions. Since then, they have spread out to urban areas. Between 2005 and 2013, the number of NPs in Canada quadrupled rising from 825 to 3 477, with most working either in primary care or in hospital (Canadian Institute for Health Information, 2014). Although all provinces and territories now have legislation in place authorising their practice, most NPs (about 60%) work in one province only (the province of Ontario, which is the most populated province).

The number of students admitted in NP programmes increased rapidly between 2002 and 2009, from about 150 in 2002 up to 450 in 2009 and 2010, fuelling the recent growth in the number of NPs in Canada (Figure 3.12). The number subsequently dropped in 2011, possibly linked to a re-organisation of education programmes at that time. While NP programmes used to be offered at three different levels (post-RN diploma, master's degree and post-master's degree), there was a move in 2011 to harmonise the educational requirement, with a master's degree becoming the norm. This may have prompted some students to delay their applications to see what would be the final arrangement regarding the educational requirement (Canadian Nurses Association and Canadian Association of Schools of Nursing, 2013).

In the Netherlands, more than 1 300 NPs were employed in 2012 up from less than 200 in 2005. A two-year master's degree is required to become a NP in the Netherlands. Between 2005 and 2012, the number of students admitted in the nine universities offering these programmes increased from 220 to 350, with a large increase in 2012 (Figure 3.13).

The Dutch Ministry of Health, Welfare and Sports indicated in 2013 that it will continue to encourage the intake of students in NP programmes (as well as in programmes to train PAs), as a strategy to ensure a sufficient number of primary care providers. This pro-active training policy is complemented by a plan to strengthen the roles and responsibilities of NPs in the primary care sector (De Bruijn-Geraets, 2014). Contrary to the experience in the United States and Canada, only about 10% of NPs in the Netherlands worked in primary care in 2012. To strengthen their role in primary care, the education and training curricula of NPs will be reinforced in primary care delivery. In addition, in 2012, the scope of practice of NPs in primary care was expanded to include the prescription of certain drugs and the possibility to conduct diagnosis and prescribe treatments for some patients. GPs who wish to contribute to NPs training and recruitment can also receive financial support to do so (Freund et al., 2015).

Figure 3.12. Admissions to nurse practitioner programmes, Canada, 2002-11

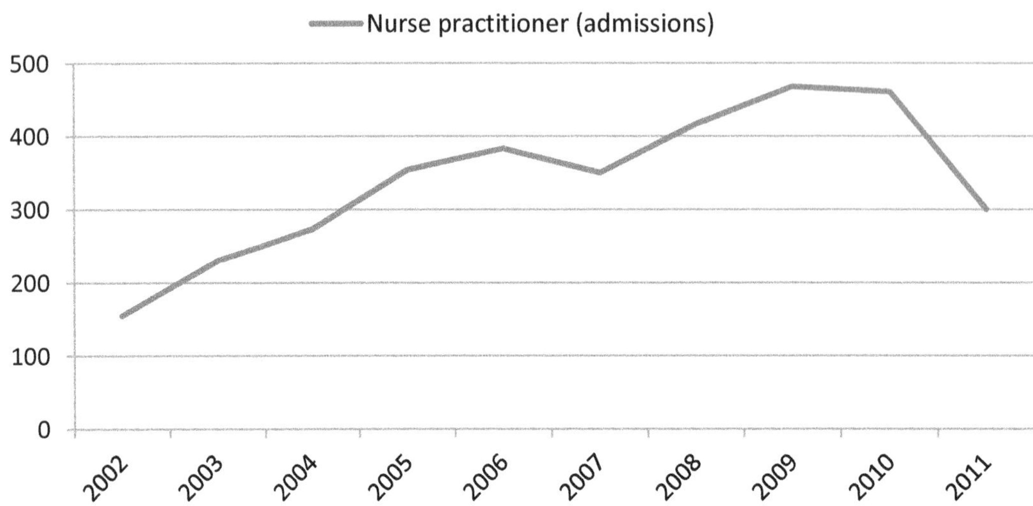

Source: CNA – Canadian Nurses Association and CASN – Canadian Association of Schools of Nursing (2013), *Registered Nurses Education in Canada Statistics 2011-12*, Ottawa.

StatLink http://dx.doi.org/10.1787/888933326229

Figure 3.13. Admissions to nurse practitioner programmes, the Netherlands, 2005-12

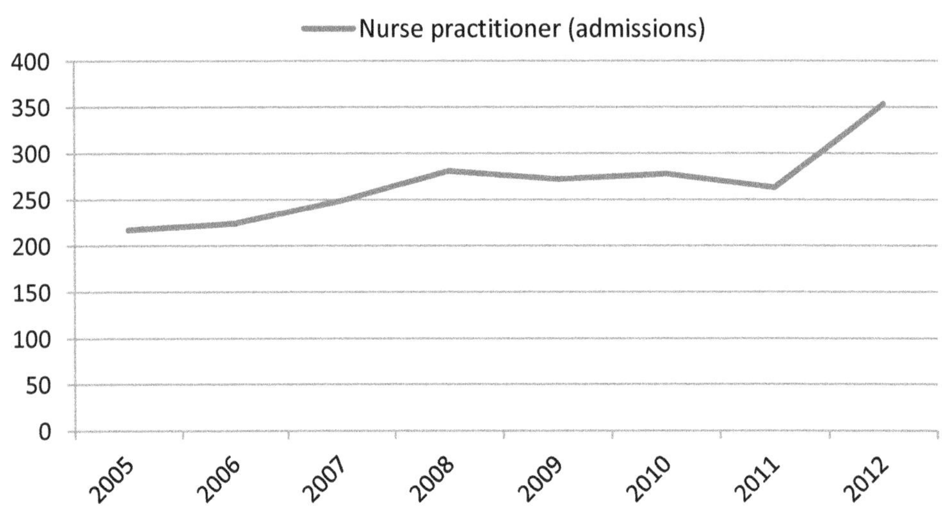

Source: ACMMP – Advisory Committee on Medical Manpower Planning (2013), *The 2013 Recommendations for Medical Specialist Training*, Capaciteitsorgaan, Utrecht.

StatLink http://dx.doi.org/10.1787/888933326239

The growing role and deployment of NPs in various countries will ultimately depend on the share of health services they are able to provide in primary care or in hospital. Past experience shows that NPs' roles and responsibilities tend to expand more easily in times and places that are underserved by doctors.

3.6. Conclusions

Changes to domestic admissions in medical and nursing education and training programmes is a key policy lever governments can use to adjust the supply of doctors and nurses to projected demand. Since the 1970s, most OECD countries have implemented some form of *numerus clausus* policies to regulate entry in medical education, and many countries have also extended the use of this policy to control entry in nursing education and other health-related programmes. The main rationale for setting a *numerus clausus* was and remains to control public spending for these education and training programmes, to limit entry to the most able applicants and to avoid any over-supply which may generate additional spending pressures through supply-induced demand. The rationale for a *numerus clausus* is generally stronger for medical education than for nursing education, given the longer duration and higher public cost of training new doctors and the greater risks of supply-induced demand. Such a rationale justified, for example, the government decision in Australia a few years ago to abandon a *numerus clausus* in nursing education and many other university programmes, but to keep such control on entry into medical education.

Although *numerus clausus* policies have been in place for several decades now, their legitimacy and management have regularly been criticised. *Numerus clausus* limit students' freedom to pursue higher education and the freedom of universities to offer more training places. It is also difficult for governments to set the "right quotas", which are inevitably based on future projections of supply and demand of different occupational groups that are fraught with uncertainty. In many countries, *numerus clausus* policies have often been characterised by "bust and boom" cycles, with periods of tight controls of student intakes to avoid any over-supply followed by periods of large increases to respond to real or perceived shortages of doctors or nurses.

This chapter reviewed changes in *numerus clausus* policies in a number of OECD countries since 2000. Across a majority of OECD countries, the number of students admitted in medical and nursing education programmes has increased substantially in response to concerns of shortages and a recognition in some countries of the need to become more "self-sufficient" and rely less on foreign-trained doctors and nurses. But there have been variations in the timing and size of this expansion. Following a period of strong growth in the early 2000s, some countries have stabilised around the mid-2000s entry in medical education programmes at the new higher level (e.g., Finland, France, the Netherlands and the United Kingdom), whereas in other countries the number of students continued to grow throughout the period (e.g., Australia, Canada and New Zealand). There were also variations in the timing and rate of growth in nursing education. In some countries, nursing education admissions increased mostly in the early 2000s (e.g. France), whereas there was a steady increase in other countries (e.g., Australia, Finland and the United States).

How to determine what may be the right level of student intakes that may be sufficient to meet projected future demand while avoiding any excessive production of new doctors and nurses which would result in a waste of money and human capital and make it more difficult to achieve any desirable change in the scope of practice of different providers? This is a question that many governments have struggled with and will continue to struggle with in the coming years, given the wide range of factors that are affecting the future demand and supply of various categories of health workers and the uncertainties regarding how these factors will evolve. These uncertainties call for a regular re-assessment of current and future health labour market conditions to adjust *numerus clausus* policies accordingly, but without overreacting to cyclical factors that may only have passing effects.

There is evidence in some OECD countries that the steady growth in student intakes and graduation rates over the past decade may be exceeding current and projected demand. Some recent medical and nursing graduates are facing difficulties finding jobs, indicating a current over-supply. The change in the future outlook of the nurse workforce in the United States provides a striking example of how a large increase in student intakes, sustained over many years, can address any projected shortages and possibly lead to an over-supply. Whereas the US Department of Health and Human Services had projected in 2004 that there might be a shortage of about 1 million registered nurses (RNs) by 2020 if training rates were to continue at their level of 2001, the number of students admitted in RN education programmes doubled between 2001 and 2013, rising from about 100 000 to 200 000 per year. Training 100 000 more RNs per year over ten years results in 1 million additional RNs. The most recent projections from the US Department of Health and Human Services is that if student admission rates remain at their 2013 level, there might be an over-supply of more than 300 000 RNs by 2025. There might still be shortages in some States or local regions, but the overall supply would be more than sufficient to meet the demand if it is well distributed (HHS, 2014).

In countries where admissions in medical education have increased quite rapidly over the past decade, there is a need to ensure proper co-ordination between the number of new medical graduates and the number of post-graduate training places available, or else some medical graduates will simply not have the opportunity to complete their specialty training, leading to a waste of public and private resources. This "bottleneck" issue has come up in Australia and the United States, where there are strong pressures to open up a greater number of post-graduate training places to allow more medical graduates to complete their training, but at the risk of possibly ending up training too many new doctors which might have serious cost implications.

Some countries, like Canada, France and the United States, have recently opted to increase the number of post-graduate training places in general medicine to try to achieve a better balance between generalists and specialists. In France, the number of post-graduate training places in general medicine has increased more rapidly than places in other medical or surgical specialties over the past decade, reaching a ratio of almost 1:1. However, for these policies to be fully effective and have long lasting effects in the composition of the medical workforce, they need to be complemented by other measures to make general medicine more attractive financially and in other aspects of working conditions.

Some countries, such as Canada, the Netherlands and the United States, have also taken steps to increase training programmes for advanced practice nurses such as nurse practitioners (NPs). One of the goals is to respond to growing needs for primary care workers and possible shortages of GPs through increasing the supply of other "mid-level" providers. The United States and Canada have led the way in creating the first training programmes for advanced practice nurses back in the 1960s, with some other countries following through since then. The United States is the country where the number and share of NPs among all nurses is the highest, with NPs now representing more than 5% of all RNs. This growing number has been fuelled by steady increases in admissions and graduations from NP programmes, with the number of NP graduates more than doubling over the past decade. The US experience provides an example of the potential scope for development of NPs in other countries.

Proper management of *numerus clausus* policies for medical and nursing education needs to be based on more robust health workforce data and health workforce planning models that take into account the interactions between different health care providers and are regularly updated. Box 3.4 summarises some of the main recommendations from a 2013 OECD review of health workforce planning models.

Box 3.4. Recommendations to improve health workforce planning in OECD countries

- **Health workforce planning is not an exact science and needs regular updating:** Assessing the future supply and demand for doctors, nurses or other health professionals 10 or 15 years down the road is a complex task, fraught with uncertainties on the supply side and even more so on the demand side. Projections are inevitably based on a set of assumptions about the future; these assumptions need to be regularly re-assessed in light of changing circumstances, new data, and the effect of new policies and programmes.

- **Need to know first where we are before we can know where we're heading:** The first step of any good health workforce projection is good data about the current situation. One of the main benefits of strengthening health workforce planning efforts is that it often triggers improvements in this crucial first step.

- **Health workforce projections should help avoid a "yo-yo" approach to student intakes and entry into medical and nursing occupations:** Available evidence shows that employment in the health sector tends to be less sensitive to economic cycles than employment in other sectors, and there is also a long time lag between decisions about medical student intakes and when these students will actually enter the labour market. Hence, health workforce planning should keep an eye on long-term structural factors and avoid being overly sensitive to cyclical fluctuations.

- **Supply-side improvements need to focus more on retirement patterns:** Most health workforce projection models have focused their attention on new entry into different professions, but have paid less attention to exit through retirement. There is a need to consider more closely the complex issue of work-to-retirement patterns, particularly for doctors but also for other professions, as a large number of health care providers are approaching the "standard" retirement age and their retirement decisions will have a major impact on supply in the coming years.

- **Need to move from uni-professional to multi-professional health workforce planning:** Health workforce projection models need to be able to assess in a more integrated way the impact of different health care delivery models, as many countries are looking at ways to re-organise the delivery of services to better respond to population ageing and the growing burden of chronic diseases. Moving from uni-professional to multi-professional approaches to health workforce planning is particularly important in the primary care sector where the roles and responsibilities of different providers (doctors, nurses and other providers) is rapidly evolving in some countries.

- **Health workforce planning models need to address adequately the geographic distribution of health workers:** Any nationwide balance of health workers does not necessarily mean that regional shortages or surpluses do not exist. A proper assessment of gaps between supply and demand needs to go below the national level to assess the geographic distribution of health workers, and how this might evolve over time under different scenarios.

Source: Ono, T., G. Lafortune and M. Schoenstein (2013), "Health Workforce Planning in OECD Countries: A Review of 26 Projection Models from 18 Countries", *OECD Health Working Papers No. 62*, OECD Publishing, Paris, http://dx.doi.org/10.1787/5k44t787zcwb-en.

Recognising the need to strengthen workforce planning, the European Commission has funded a *Joint Action on Health Workforce Planning and Forecasting*. This Joint Action is set-up as a group of European experts that analyse future skills and competences in the health sector and inform countries on challenges and best practices on health workforce planning and forecasting. One of the main outputs of this Joint Action has been a handbook on health workforce planning methodologies across EU countries.

An increasingly important factor challenging the setting of a *numerus clausus* at the national level is the growing internationalisation of medical and nursing education and of health labour markets more generally. The growing international mobility of medical and nursing students and health workers makes it more difficult to determine, at a national level, how many students should be trained to respond to any projected demand. The Netherlands provides a good example of how this added layer of complexity and uncertainty may affect health workforce planning. In 2010, the Netherlands decided to increase the *numerus clausus* for medical education under the assumption that there would be a reduction in incoming foreign-trained doctors. However, this reduction did not occur. Following a re-assessment of the supply and demand situation three years later, the decision was made to reverse this earlier decision and return to the training level that existed up to 2010. While getting reliable data on migration patterns and making realistic projections about future developments is not easy, countries increasingly need to take into account in their health workforce planning models the inflows of foreign-trained doctors and nurses, as well as the outflows of doctors and nurses (those moving outside the country), in order to be able to assess more precisely domestic training needs.

One factor hindering health workforce policies in general and *numerus clausus* policies more specifically is weak governance and management arrangements. In several OECD countries, *numerus clausus* policies are still based on weak evidence and opaque decision-making processes. The Netherlands is an exception, as it has strengthened the governance and management structure of its *numerus clausus* policy for medical education (as well as dentistry education). Following a period of prolonged doctor shortages, the Dutch Government decided in 2000 to create the Advisory Council on Medical Manpower Planning (ACMMP), an independent health workforce planning agency composed by professionals, educational institutions and health insurance companies, with a mandate to formulate and agree on a set of recommendations for student quotas entering medicine. These recommendations are based on a solid health workforce planning model developed and maintained by the Dutch Institute of Health Service Research (NIVEL). The recommendations from this Committee are then used by the Dutch Government to decide on the number of students that should be admitted in medical education and training programmes. Since its establishment 15 years ago, this governance structure – within the Dutch context – has significantly improved the decision-making process based on solid evidence and engagement of all relevant stakeholders and has helped to reduce any mismatches between physician demand and supply (Van Greuningen et al., 2012). In many other OECD countries, the governance of *numerus clausus* policies needs to be strengthened.

Notes

1. The authors would like to thank Ian Brownwood (from the OECD Health Division) and Caroline Hager and Leon van Berkel (from the European Commission) for many useful comments.

2. One special feature of the *numerus clausus* policy in France is that student selection is made only after the first year of medical studies (which has now been broadened to be a first year of studies in health, known as *Première Année Commune aux Études de Santé)* through a national exam (*concours*). In 2010/11, only around 20% of first-year students interested in pursuing medical education were able to move on to the second year (ONDPS, 2015).

3. The EU Directive on the recognition of professional qualifications (Directive 2005/36/EC, which was replaced more recently by Directive 2013/55/EU) allows the automatic recognition of qualifications for certain professions, including doctors and nurses trained in another EU country.

4. These refer only to allopathic medical schools. In addition, new osteopathic medical schools have also opened in recent years, also contributing to the increase in student admissions.

5. In most OECD countries, general medicine is now recognised as a specialty in its own right giving it the same prestige as other medical or surgical specialties, thereby blurring the distinction between "generalist" and "specialist" training. In this section training in general medicine is distinguished from training in other specialties.

6. Interestingly, a 2013 survey of physicians in Canada sought their views about which specialty areas would be expanding in the coming years. Geriatric medicine ranked first, with more than 90% of physicians foreseeing that this specialty would be growing in the future, followed by dermatology, emergency medicine, psychiatry and neurosurgery (Buske, 2014). But despite this expected growth in the demand for geriatric medicine, the number of post-graduate trainees in geriatric medicine in 2013 remained very low and much lower than in paediatrics (CAPER, 2014).

7. In the United States, both family medicine and internal medicine doctors are considered as generalists, given that there are several similarities in their practice. Nonetheless, there remain differences in terms of patient groups (internal medicine doctors usually only consult adults and elderly people, whereas family medicine doctors also take care of children and adolescents) and areas of specialisation (for example, internal medicine doctors can sub-specialise in cardiology or pulmonology).

8. This section focusses on education programmes for NPs as this is one of the largest categories of recognised advanced practice nurses in several countries. Nonetheless other programmes exist to train advanced or specialised nurses. For example, in the United States, a variety of master's programmes are available to train clinical nurse specialists (who account for about 20% of all advanced practice nurses), nurse anaesthetists (accounting for about 13% of APNs) and nurse midwives (7% of APNs) (Institute of Medicine, 2011).

References

AAFP – American Academy of Family Physicians (2014), *Family Physician Workforce Reform – Recommendations of the American Academy of Family Physicians*, Kansas.

AAMC – Association of American Medical Colleges (2012), *A Snapshot of the New and Developing Medical Schools in the U.S. and Canada*, AAMC, Washington D.C.

AAMC (2006), *Statement of the Physician Workforce*, AAMC, Washington D.C.

AANP – American Association of Nurse Practitioners (2015), "NP Fact Sheet", available at www.aanp.org.

AANP (2013), "NP Fact Sheet", available at www.aanp.org.

ACMMP – Advisory Committee on Medical Manpower Planning (2013), *The 2013 Recommendations for Medical Specialist Training*, Capaciteitsorgaan, Utrecht.

ACMMP (2010), *The 2010 Recommendations for Medical Specialist Training*, Capaciteitsorgaan, Utrecht.

ANMF – Australian Nursing and Midwifery Federation (2014), "Submission to the 457 Integrrity Review", Australian Nursing and Midwifery Federation Journals, Kingston.

Auerbach, D. et al. (2013), "The Nursing Workforce in an Era of Health Care Reform", *New England Journal of Medicine*, Vol. 368, No. 16, pp. 1470-1472.

Bradley, D. et al. (2008), *Review of Australian Higher Education: Final Report*, Department of Education and Training, Australian Government.

Buske, L. (2014), *Demand for Physicians and their Services*, Canadian Collaborative Centre for Physician Resources, Canadian Medical Association.

CNA – Canadian Nurses Association and CASN – Canadian Association of Schools of Nursing (2013), *Registered Nurses Education in Canada Statistics 2011-12*, Ottawa.

CAPER – Canada's Definitive Source of Data on Post M.D. Training (2014), "Field of Post-M.D. Training by Faculty of Medicine Providing Post-M.D. Training 2013-2014", database available at http://www.caper.ca.

Chenot, J. (2009), "Undergraduate Medical Education in Germany", German Medical Science, Vol. 7.

CIHI – Canadian Institute for Health Information (2014), *Regulated Nurses, 2013*, Ottawa.

Creed, P., J. Searle and M. Rogers (2010), "Medical Specialty Prestige and Lifestyle Preferences for Medical Students", *Journal of Social Science and Medicine*, Vol. 71, No. 6, pp. 1084-1088.

De Bruijn-Geraets, D. (2014), "Evaluating Newly Acquired Authority of Nurse Practitioners and Physician Assistants for Reserved Medical Procedures in the Netherlands: A Study Protocol", *Journal of Advanced Nursing*, Vol. 70, No. 11, pp. 2673-2682.

Delamaire, M. and G. Lafortune (2010), "Nurses in Advanced Roles: A Description and Evaluation of Experiences in 12 Developed Countries", *OECD Health Working Papers*, No. 54, OECD Publishing, Paris, http://dx.doi.org/10.1787/5kmbrcfms5g7-en.

Department of Health (2012), "The Health and Education National Strategic Exchange – Review of Medical and Dental School Intakes in England", UK Government.

DREES (2014), "Les affectations des étudiants en médecine à l'issue des épreuves classantes nationales en 2013", *Études et Résultats*, No. 894, Paris.

DREES (2011), "Les affectations des étudiants en médecine à l'issue des épreuves classantes nationales en 2010", Études et Résultats, No. 767.

European Federation of Nurses Associations (2012), "Caring in Crisis: The Impact of the Financial Crisis on Nurses and Nursing – A Comparative Overview of 34 European Countries", Brussels.

Freund, T. et al. (2015), "Skill Mix, Roles and Remuneration in the Primary Care Workforce: Who Are the Healthcare Professionals in the Primary Care Teams Across the World?", *International Journal of Nursing Studies*, Vol. 52, No. 3, pp. 727-743.

General Medical Council (2014), *A Reference Guide for Postgraduate Specialty Training in the UK*, London.

Harris, J.E. et al. (2013), "Specialty Choice in Times of Economic Crisis: A Cross-sectional Survey of Spanish Medical Students", *BMJ Open*, Vol. 3, No. 2.

Hawthorne, L. (2012), "Health Workforce Migration to Australia – Policy Trends and Outcomes 2004 to 2010", University of Melbourne, Melbourne.

Health and Human Services (2014), "The Future of the Nursing Workforce: National- and State-level Projections, 2012-2025", US Department of Health and Human Resources, Rockville, Maryland.

Health and Human Services (2013), "Projecting the Supply and Demand for Primary Care Practitioners Through 2020", US Department of Health and Human Resources, Rockville, Maryland.

Health and Human Services, Health Resources and Services Administration (2004), "What Is Behind HRSA's Projected Supply, Demand, and Shortage of Registered Nurses?, Washington, D.C.

Health Resources and Services Administration (2013), "Projecting the Supply and Demand for Primary Care Practitioners Through 2020", Bureau of Health Professions, National Center for Health Workforce Analysis, Health Resources and Services Administration.

Health Workforce Australia (2014), "Australia's Future Health Workforce – Nurses Detailed", Department of Health, Canberra.

Health Workforce Australia (2013), "Australia's Health Workforce Series: Nurses in Focus", Melbourne.

Health Workforce Australia (2012), "Australia's Health Workforce Series: Doctors in Focus", Melbourne.

Iglehart, J. (2013), "The Residency Mismatch", *New England Journal of Medicine*, Vol. 369, No. 4.

Institute of Medicine of the National Academies (2011), *The Future of Nursing: Leading Change, Advancing Health*, Washington D.C.

Joyce C., J. Stoelwinder and L. Piterman (2007), "Riding the Wave: Current and Emerging Trends in Graduates from Australian University Medical Schools", *Medical Journal of Australia*, Vol. 186, No. 6, pp. 309-312.

Kemp D. and A. Norton (2014), *Review of the Demand Driven Funding System*, Department of Education, Australian Government.

Ketel, N. et al. (2012), "The Returns to Medical School in a Regulated Labour Market: Evidence from Admission Lotteries", Faculty of Economics and Business, Amsterdam School of Economics Research Institute.

Malgeri, A., P. Michelutti and M. Van Hoegaerden (2015), *Handbook on Health Workforce Planning Methodologies Across EU Countries*, Ministry of Health of the Slovak Republic.

Medical Careers (2014), "Postgraduate Doctors", www.medicalcareers.nhs.uk/postgraduate_doctors.

Miani, C. et al. (2015), *Best Practice: Medical Training from an International Perspective*, Rand Corporation

Mirvis, D. (2013), "Choosing a Medical Specialty: The Difference Between What Students Want and What Society Needs", *Journal of Health Policy Research*, Vol. 2, No. 18.

NHS (2014), "Securing the Future GP Workforce Delivering the Mandate on GP Expansion – GP Taskforce Final Report", Department of Health, UK Government.

Ono, T., G. Lafortune and M. Schoenstein (2013), "Health Workforce Planning in OECD Countries: A Review of 26 Projection Models from 18 Countries", *OECD Health Working Papers No. 62*, OECD Publishing, Paris, http://dx.doi.org/10.1787/5k44t787zcwb-en.

ONDPS – Observatoire national de la démographie des professions de santé (2015), "Rapport 2013-2014: La régulation démographique des professionnels de santé par les flux d'étudiants, la situation démographique des chirurgiens-dentistes, bilan de la filiarisation", Paris.

Petterson. S. et al. (2012), "Projecting US Primary Care Physician Workforce Needs: 2012-2025", *Annals of Family Medicine*, Vol. 10, No. 6, pp. 503-509.

Pong, R. (2012), "Post-M.D. Training in Family Medicine in Canada: Continuity and Change over a 15-year period", Ottawa.

Santana, P., H. Peixoto and N. Duarte (2014), "Demography of Physicians in Portugal: Prospective Analysis", *Acta Médica Portuguesa*, Vol. 27, No. 2, pp. 246-251.

Spitzer, A. and B. Perrenoud (2006), "Reforms in Nursing Education Across Western Europe: Implementation Processes and Current Status", *Journal of Professional Nursing*, Vol. 22, No. 3, pp. 162-171.

Van Greuningen, M., R.S. Batenburg, L.F.J Van der Velden (2012), "Ten Years of Health Workforce Planning in the Netherlands: A Tentative Evaluation of GP Planning as an Example", *Human Resources for Health*, Vol. 10, No. 1:21, BioMed Central, London, http://www.human-resources-health.com/content/10/1/21.

Annex 3.A1
Medical and nursing education and training programmes pathways in OECD countries

Medical education and training

Over the past decades, the education and training pathways for students in medicine have become increasingly diversified in most OECD countries, with more possible entry points for prospective students and "passerelles" (bridges) between fields of studies, as well as greater choices to specialise in various fields in post-graduate training programmes.

Figure 3.A1.1 shows a few of the most common pathways in initial medical education and post-graduate training in different OECD countries. In some countries, such as the United States, medical education is offered mainly as a graduate degree, following completion of a first bachelor degree in biology or other fields. In other countries, such as France, medical education comes in the form of an undergraduate degree, with students accessing medicine directly from secondary education. Some other countries offer a hybrid model of medical education, with possibilities to enter both at the undergraduate and/or graduate levels for eligible students. For instance, in the United Kingdom, while the majority of students still access medicine right from secondary school (undergraduate degree), since 2000, some universities accept students with background in life sciences, dentistry or biomedicine, into the third year (the start of a graduate degree). These additional entries into medical education programmes were designed to enlarge access to students who hold a bachelor in a relevant field.

Once a student completes basic medical education, he/she typically has to take a final exam which might serve to validate his/her degree, rank them for their post-graduate training and, in some cases, also grant them with a medical license (often accompanied with some conditions regarding their scope of practice). The following step is usually some specialty training through some forms of internship or residency period. Each country offers various medical specialties of different lengths. Generally, training to become a Family Doctor/General Practitioner (GP) is one of the shortest specialties, averaging three years in many countries. Other specialisations, notably surgery, take longer. In the United States, residency programmes usually last on average three to eight years, but if a student decides to pursue a more advanced sub-specialty, the training can prolong up to eleven years. In some countries, an initial training of one to two years (normally in hospital) precedes any specialty training. For instance, in the United Kingdom, a two-year post-graduate training (called "foundation training") was introduced right after medical school in 2005 (Medical Careers, 2014). During this training period, new graduates rotate, every 3 to 4 months, between different specialities. The first year leads to registration with the General Medical Council. The completion of the second year allows the trainee to apply for specialty training programmes (General Medical Council, 2014).

In most countries, the number of specialties and subspecialties in post-graduate training programmes has increased over time. For example, in Canada, the number of fields of specialisation in post-graduate training has increased from 76 in 1996/97 to 86 in 2013/14 (CAPER, 2014).

Figure 3.A1.1. Models of entry into medical education and post-graduate training

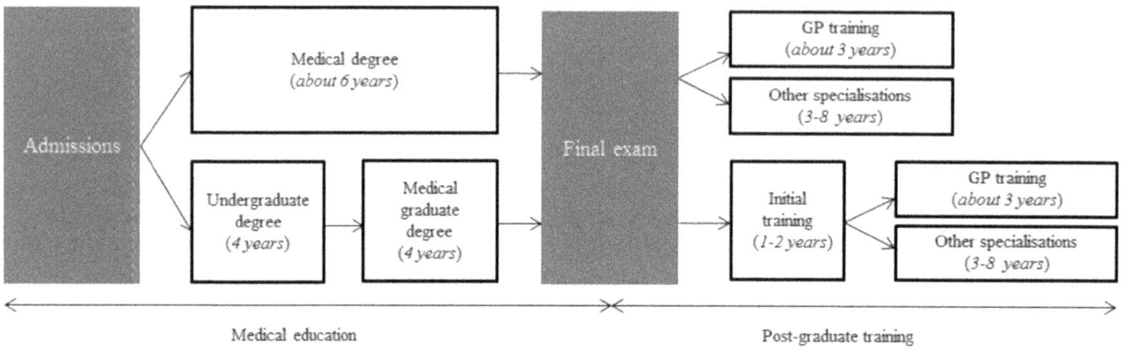

Nursing education and training

Across OECD countries, there are also several models for initial, specialised and advanced nursing education (Figure 3.A1.2). During the 1980s, with the developments in health services and increased complexity of care, in many OECD countries, nurse education shifted from hospital based training programmes to university based degrees. This led to a new era of nurse education, allowing nurses to not only access undergraduate, but also post-graduate level education. In Europe, over the last three decades, there have been two main phases of reform to harmonise nurse education. Firstly, by creating a unified European platform of nursing programmes and licencing, to improve the level of graduates, and allow mutual recognition across EU countries. Secondly, to integrate nursing programmes within higher education systems and have university based degrees (Spitzer and Perrenoud, 2006).

Figure 3.A1.2. Models of entry to basic nursing education and more advanced education paths

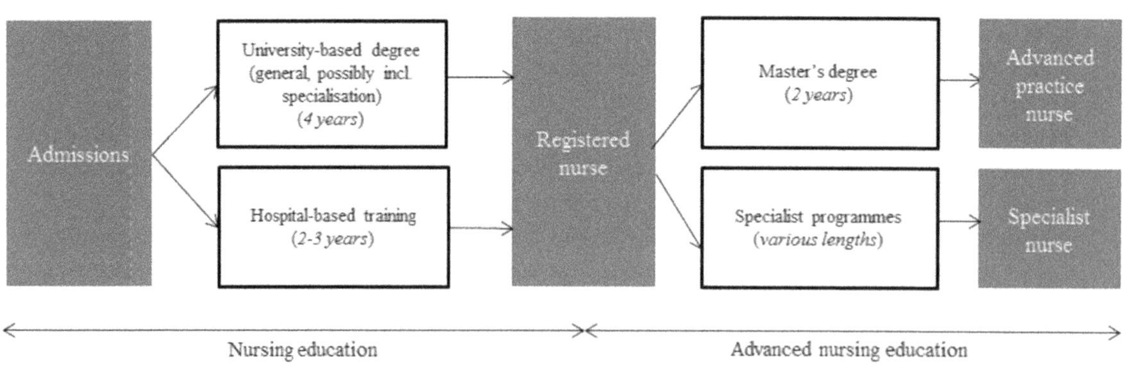

Following their first university degree, nurses have numerous options for more advanced studies or specialisation. For example, in certain countries, nurses can opt for more advanced studies (e.g., a master's degree) to become an Advanced Practice Nurse (APN) such as a Nurse Practitioner. In the United States, a range of master's degrees are available to prepare students for an array of different positions as APNs such as NPs, Clinical Nurse Specialists, Clinical Nurse Leaders, among others. PhD programmes can be also pursued after a master's degree and are usually more research oriented (Institute of Medicine, 2011).

Registered nurses can also further enhance their professional knowledge and scope of practice by choosing a specialty programme. A wide variety of programmes may be available in each country. In the United Kingdom, four main tracks are predominant: clinical, management, education and research. For each one of these options, several career options exist depending on the level of education the student reaches. Whereas a postgraduate degree might allow for a career as a nurse consultant, a PhD would open the option to become a professor at University.

Annex 3.A2
Trends in graduates from medical and nursing education programmes in OECD countries

Changes in *numerus clausus* policies in medical and nursing education programmes can also be assessed by looking at the number of graduates from these programmes. The number of graduates can serve as a proxy to measure decisions on admissions a few years earlier. However, trends in graduation rates may also be influenced by any changes in dropout rates during these studies. Given that completing a medical or nursing education programme takes several years, the number of graduates will reflect decisions on *numerus clausus* taken several years earlier (about 5 to 6 years in the case of medical education and about 3 to 4 years for nursing education), as well as the dropout rates of students during these programmes.

Data on the number of graduates from medical and nursing education programmes are available for nearly all OECD countries, based on national responses to the OECD/Eurostat/WHO Joint Questionnaire on non-monetary health care statistics. Table 3.A2.1 shows the trends in number of graduates from medical education programmes in OECD countries between 2005 and 2013. In most OECD countries, the number of graduates has increased between 2005 and 2013, with the growth rate being particularly strong in Australia, Finland, France, Poland and Portugal, reflecting the strong rise in admission rates five to six years earlier. There has also been a strong rise in the number of medical graduates in Slovenia and Belgium. On the other hand, the increase has been much more modest in Italy, Japan and Sweden. Austria and Korea are the only countries where the number of medical graduates has decreased between 2005 and 2013. In Korea, these numbers are not expected to grow significantly in the coming years given that student intakes in medical education programmes have remained fairly stable between 2007 and 2012.

As is the case for medical graduates, the number of nursing graduates has also increased in most of OECD countries from 2005 to 2013. This increase has been particularly strong in countries such as Chile, Mexico, Poland and Turkey (Table 3.A2.2). In Poland, the number of nursing graduates increased from about 7 000 in 2006 to over 13 500 in 2013. The growth rate has been much slower in Austria (virtually nil or even slightly declining).

Table 3.A2.1. Trends in number of graduates from medical education programmes, OECD countries, 2005-13

	2005	2006	2007	2008	2009	2010	2011	2012	2013
Australia	1 798	1 884	2 117	2 389	2 361	2 662	3 011	3 179	3 573
Austria	1 569	1 456	1 835	1 814	1 726	1 466	1 413	1 170	..
Belgium	763	681	732	758	851	980	1 125	1 180	1 176
Canada	1 878	1 957	2 047	2 122	2 339	2 449	2 533	2 641	2 662
Chile	746	750	664	815	1 101	936	1,077	1,355	1,036
Czech Republic	1 069	1 041	1 108	1 163	1 319	1 458	1 460	1 591	1 338
Denmark	1 152	1 122	1 192	1 121	1 204	1 210	1 179	1 039	1 032
Estonia	106	128	106	112	120	149	125	147	144
Finland	337	395	367	546	500	603	621	790	624
France	3 441	3 354	3 843	4 202	4 429	4 689	5 646	5 883	..
Germany	8 870	8 724	9 574	9 857	10 069	9 894	9 572	9 587	9 801
Greece	1 472	1 635	1 599	..	..	..	..	..	..
Hungary	1 151	1 069	1 005	960	923	1 040	1 148	1 374	1 496
Iceland	44	40	36	49	37	44	44	49	..
Ireland	594	641	726	673	722	785	738	781	931
Israel	312	310	296	325	300	314	377	304	408
Italy	6 415	6 143	6 816	6 796	6 682	6 732	6 699	6 631	6 735
Japan	7 392	7 639	7 647	7 434	7 561	7 619	7 631	7 501	7 639
Korea	4 363	3 973	4 354	4 454	4 449	4 064	3 992	4 096	4 009
Mexico	11 638	10 619	11 936	12 912	12 631	12 812	13 231	13 618	11 716
Netherlands	1 756	1 842	2 019	2 022	2 075	2 276	2 456	2 467	2 422
New Zealand	297	287	284	308	337	317	351	348	379
Norway	467	461	497	496	516	551	568	619	578
Poland	2 349	2 308	2 550	2 727	2 788	3 081	3 349	3 549	3 757
Portugal	736	812	1 029	1 101	1 126	1 262	1 287	1 394	1 426
Slovak Republic	557	509	535	458	421	577	590	621	690
Slovenia	162	128	129	174	162	229	206	266	245
Spain	4 064	3 951	3 841	3 922	3 882	4 299	4 199	4 457	4 770
Sweden	805	910	932	950	993	969	1 010	1 126	986
Switzerland	622	594	612	667	729	813	744	782	786
Turkey	4 494	4 532	4 899	4 872	4 753	5 087	5 138	4 981	4 949
United Kingdom	6 820	7 390	7 520	8 115	8 210	8 490	8 435	8 840	8 450
United States	18 516	18 635	19 140	19 532	20 555	20 469	21 522	21 799	22 963

Note: There is no data for Luxembourg as there is no medical school in that country.

The statistical data for Israel are supplied by and under the responsibility of the relevant Israeli authorities. The use of such data by the OECD is without prejudice to the status of the Golan Heights, East Jerusalem and Israeli settlements in the West Bank under the terms of international law.

Source: OECD Health Statistics 2015 (the database includes the underlying sources in each country).

StatLink http://dx.doi.org/10.1787/888933326247

Table 3.A2.2. Trends in number of graduates from nursing education programmes, OECD countries, 2005-13

	2005	2006	2007	2008	2009	2010	2011	2012	2013
Australia	..	..	..	13 096	13 782	14 886	16 005	16 318	17 306
Austria	..	4 758	4 898	4 890	4 006	4 662	4 813	4 598	..
Belgium	4 147	3 324	3 566	3 476	4 022	4 542	4 140	4 735	5 305
Canada	..	..	15 489	14 928	15 221	16 831	18 858	19 340	19 144
Chile	2 474	2 760	2 438	2 840	4 932	7 061	6 436	6 939	7 705
Czech Republic	4 843	5 029	3 643	1 612	1 457	1 283	1 822	1 810	1 565
Denmark	4 393	4 555	4 627	4 984	4 597	5 214	5 348	5 167	..
Estonia	483	470	591	377	472	418	456	463	479
Finland	2 349	2 453	2 633	2 981	3 076	3 368	3 430	3 594	3 747
France	20 982	20 982	21 648	21 566	22 122	22 311	23 113	26 447	25 619
Germany	36 588	38 155	37 499	35 877	36 968	36 860	36 959	42 256	44 620
Hungary	4 213	4 031	3 684	3 158	3 369	2 863	2 544	2 596	3 364
Iceland	200	276	224	327	206	248	208	224	..
Ireland	1 425	1 508	1 410	1 572	1 440	1 641	1 720	1 518	1 528
Israel	1 150	1 080	1 009	957	860	848	879	1 109	1 271
Italy	9 046	9 388	10 491	10 091	10 821	9 776	11 389	12 153	13 860
Japan	44 852	45 805	46 253	47 704	46 968	48 740	49 429	50 158	52 058
Korea	..	29 600	32 224	35 099	38 293	45 268	46 997	45 889	48 861
Luxembourg	90	89	88	81	89	101	130	130	61
Mexico	5 051	5 655	7 046	7 265	9 175	10 879	11 492	12 336	12 752
Netherlands	5 406	5 562	5 876	6 181	6 323	6 519	6 338	6 222	6 302
New Zealand	1 310	1 403	1 318	1 372	1 343	1 454	1 522	1 627	1 966
Norway	3 652	3 593	3 696	3 282	3 488	3 200	3 347	3 522	3 653
Poland	..	6 938	7 918	9 187	8 428	9 653	17 323	12 395	13 561
Portugal	2 954	3 457	3 594	3 571	3 792	3 706	3 391	3 005	2 666
Slovak Republic	1 731	3 732	..	2 713	3 061	3 167	3 159	3 430	3 416
Slovenia	1 480	1 723	1 788	1 711	1 641	1 665	1 679	1 614	1 598
Spain	8 699	8 764	8 748	8 987	9 472	10 098	11 654	8 194	8 783
Switzerland	4 540	4 549	4 960	5 124	5 738	5 983	6 180	5 699	6 759
Turkey	5 386	5 709	7 001	3 927	4 288	11 597	14 046	14 865	..
United Kingdom	19 982	20 940	21 388	20 398e	18 268e	20 666e	21 606e	23 412e	27 006e
United States	149 501	164 190	173 495	185 801	194 575	201 611	202 692	208 495e	200 341e

Note: e stands for estimated figure.

The statistical data for Israel are supplied by and under the responsibility of the relevant Israeli authorities. The use of such data by the OECD is without prejudice to the status of the Golan Heights, East Jerusalem and Israeli settlements in the West Bank under the terms of international law.

Source: OECD Health Statistics 2015 (the database includes the underlying sources in each country).

StatLink http://dx.doi.org/10.1787/888933326258

Annex 3.A3
Sources of data for number of students admitted to medical and nursing education

Table 3.A3.1. Sources of data for number of students admitted in medical education

	Type of source	Source name
Australia	Website	Medical Deans
Austria	Website	STATcube, Statistical Database of Statistics Austria, Studies at public universities
Belgium	Contact through email	Executive Office Education and Training
Canada	Website	Association of Faculties of Medicine of Canada
Finland	Contact through email	Ministry of Social Affairs and Health
France	Website	DREES
Germany	Website	Statistisches Bundesamt
Ireland	Website	Higher Education Authority
Japan	Website	Ministry of Education, Culture, Sports, Science and Technology
Netherlands	Website	Advisory Committee for Medical Manpower Planning
New Zealand	Website	Medical Deans
Poland	Contact through email	Ministry of Health
Portugal	Website	Directorate General of Higher Education, Directorate General of Statistics of Education and Science
Spain	Contact through email	Ministry of Health, Social Services and Equality
Sweden	Website	Statistics Sweden
Switzerland	Website	Swiss Statistics
United Kingdom	Website	Universities and Colleges Admissions Services
United States	Website	Association of American Medical Colleges and American Association of Colleges of Osteopathic Medicine

Table 3.A3.2. Sources of data for number of students admitted in nursing education

	Type of source	Source name
Australia	Website	Higher Education Statistics, highereducationstatistics.education.gov.au
Belgium	Contact through email	Executive Office Education and Training
Canada	Website	Canadian Nurses Association/Canadian Association of Schools of Nursing
Finland	Contact through email	Ministry of Social Affairs and Health
France	Website	Ministry of Health : http://www.legifrance.gouv.fr
Netherlands	Contact through email	Kiwa.nl
Portugal	Website	Directorate General of Higher Education, Directorate General of Statistics of Education and Science
Spain	Contact through email	Ministry of Health, Social Services and Equality
United Kingdom	Website	Health Education England and Department of Health
United States	Website	National League for Nursing

Chapter 4
Trends and policies affecting the international migration of doctors and nurses to OECD countries

By Clémence Merçay (formerly from University of Neuchâtel, now with the Swiss Health Observatory),
Jean-Christophe Dumont (OECD International Migration Division)
and Gaétan Lafortune (OECD Health Division)[1]

This chapter examines recent trends in the migration of foreign-trained doctors and nurses in OECD countries and some of the policies that have affected these migration patterns. Between 2000 and 2014, the immigration of foreign-trained doctors and nurses increased in most OECD countries, although the number has generally slowed down in recent years as the number of domestically-trained doctors and nurses has steadily increased. Nevertheless, foreign-trained doctors and nurses have contributed to the overall increase in the number of doctors and nurses working in OECD countries since 2000. There have also been changes in the countries of origin of foreign-trained doctors and nurses, particularly in Europe. Some European countries that have recently become EU members and those particularly hard hit by the recession have experienced an important increase in the emigration (outflows) of their doctors and nurses to other European countries, seeking better job opportunities. While in some cases, this emigration might have helped to reduce the number of unemployed or under-employed doctors and nurses, in other cases, it exacerbated shortages of certain categories of doctors and nurses. This has prompted some countries, notably in Central and Eastern Europe, to take measures to increase the retention rates of doctors and nurses, including pay raises and improvements in working conditions.

The statistical data for Israel are supplied by and under the responsibility of the relevant Israeli authorities. The use of such data by the OECD is without prejudice to the status of the Golan Heights, East Jerusalem and Israeli settlements in the West Bank under the terms of international law.

4.1. Introduction

The international migration of doctors, nurses and other health workers is not a new phenomenon, but has drawn a lot of attention in recent years because of concerns that it might exacerbate shortages of skilled health workers in certain countries, particularly in some low-income countries that are already suffering from critical workforce shortages. The Global Code of Practice on the International Recruitment of Health Personnel, adopted by the World Health Assembly in May 2010, was designed mainly to respond to these concerns. It provides an instrument for countries to promote a more ethical recruitment of health personnel and encourage them to achieve greater "self-sufficiency" in the training of health workers, while recognising the basic human right of every person to migrate (see Box 4.1).

Box 4.1. Excerpts from the WHO Global Code of Practice on the International Recruitment of Health Personnel

Ethical international recruitment

The Code discourages the active recruitment of health care workers from developing countries with critical workforce shortages.

Equal treatment of migrant health care workers

The Code highlights the importance of equal treatment of foreign-trained health workers and their locally-trained counterparts. All health care workers should have the opportunity to assess the benefits and risks associated with employment positions, and to make informed decisions about vacancies.

Health workforce development and sustainable health systems

Member states should develop strategies for workforce planning, training and retention, adapted to the specific circumstances of each country, so that there is less of a need to recruit migrant health workers.

International co-operation

The Code encourages collaboration between health workers' countries of origin and countries of destination, so that both benefit from the migration of health professionals.

Technical collaboration and financial support

Developed countries should provide technical and financial assistance to developing countries experiencing a shortage of health workers.

Source: WHO (2010), *User's Guide to the WHO Global Code of Practice on the International Recruitment of Health Personnel.*

The 2007 OECD study on "Immigrant Health Workers in OECD Countries in the Broader Context of Highly-Skilled Migration", published in the *International Migration Outlook*, presented for the first time a complete picture of the migration flows of health personnel by countries of origin and destination (OECD, 2007). This work was recently updated in a chapter on "Changing Patterns in the International Migration of Doctors and Nurses in OECD Countries", also published in the *International Migration Outlook* (OECD, 2015). The migration patterns described in these two editions of the *International Migration Outlook* made use of population-census data to describe the number of foreign-born doctors and nurses working in OECD countries and expatriation rates from origin countries, while also including a description of foreign-trained doctors and nurses based on other (more regular) data sources.

This chapter focusses only on recent trends in the migration of foreign-trained doctors and nurses and the impact of health and migration policies on these trends. The focus on the place of training provides a more precise measure of the so-called "brain drain" issue than the place of birth (see Box 4.2). This chapter discusses the effect of changing economic conditions and institutional settings on trends in the migration of foreign-trained doctors and nurses, including the impact of the economic recession of 2008-09, the enlargement of the European Union to 13 new member states in 2004, 2007 and 2013, and the adoption of the WHO Global Code in 2010. It also discusses the impact of the growing internationalisation of higher education, which also affects medical and nursing education. While the internationalisation of medical and nursing education provides new opportunities for students to pursue their studies in another country, this is adding another layer of complexity to the monitoring of migration patterns and to policies regarding the setting of domestic education and training capacity and the capacity for some countries to absorb their domestic students who went to study abroad and wish to come back to complete their training or to work.

Box 4.2. Methods and sources to monitor the international migration of health personnel

Regular monitoring of the international migration of health personnel needs to be based on two key criteria: 1) relevancy to both countries of origin and countries of destination; and 2) feasibility of regular data collection.

Addressing the information needs for both origin and destination countries

While the migration of health workers raises concerns mainly among those countries that are losing some of their skilled workforce (the "brain drain"), statistics on *emigration* (leaving one's country of origin to settle in another) are scarce in most countries and often not reliable. This is because doctors and nurses migrating to another country generally do not have to inform their national authorities and in most cases will keep their registration in their origin country for a possible return.

Another approach to try to measure migration flows is to review information about *intention* to emigrate. All people who plan to leave their country to work as doctors or nurses in another country have to produce a certificate of good standing and proof of registration in their own country. This information can be used to estimate the emigration *potential* (the number of people who plan to leave their country). However, available evidence shows that there is a large gap between the intention to emigrate and actually doing so. This gap can be explained, for example, by difficulties in finding a job or in getting one qualification's recognised in the intended destination country.

The approach that seems the most promising and feasible in the short term to monitor health workforce migration on a regular basis is to use sources on *immigration* statistics from destination countries. Through collecting data from destination countries by country of origin and aggregating these data across destination countries, it is possible to produce estimates on the total movements of health personnel by country of origin. However, this aggregation process requires that data are available and comparable across all receiving countries, which is not always the case. Nonetheless, given that the immigration flows of health workers tend to be concentrated in a limited number of OECD destination countries, obtaining good data from these countries can go a long way towards meeting the ultimate goal of monitoring health workforce migration.

Measuring migration patterns

Migration patterns can be measured based on *nationality*, *place of birth* or *place of education/training*. The first approach, based on nationality, faces a number of shortcomings. First, foreigners disappear from the statistics when they are naturalised. Second, in several OECD countries, many people who were born and raised in a country nonetheless hold a different nationality. There is, therefore, no systematic link between migration and nationality.

Box 4.2. Methods and sources to monitor the international migration of health personnel *(cont.)*

The place of birth of doctors and nurses provides some useful information on their country of origin. However, it does not indicate when they migrated (possibly at a very young age with their parents) or where they pursued their medical or nursing education. To measure more precisely the "brain drain", the place of education and training tends to be more relevant. However, the place of education and training may over-estimate the "brain drain" if it does not properly account for the growing internationalisation of medical and nursing education – that is, people born in a country who are going to study medicine and nursing abroad, and then returning back to their origin country to practice.

Data collection approach and sources

The data presented in this chapter focus mainly on measuring the number of foreign-trained doctors and nurses who are working in OECD countries, based on both annual flows and total stocks, using the results from the 2015 OECD/Eurostat/WHO-Europe Joint Questionnaire on Non-Monetary Health Care Statistics. One of the limitations of this approach is that it has not been possible yet to identify precisely in all countries the number of these foreign-trained doctors and nurses who may be domestic residents who went to study abroad and then came back. In most countries, the main data sources are professional registries. In some countries, the data come from physician or nurse surveys. The main limitation in terms of data comparability relates to differences in the activity status of health workers. Some registries are regularly updated, making it possible to distinguish doctors and nurses who are still actively working in health systems, while other sources include all persons licensed to practise, regardless of whether they are active or not (see Annex 4.A1).

Source: Dumont, J.C., G. Lafortune and P. Zurn (2014), "Monitoring Trends in International Migration of Health Personnel: A Critical Review of Existing Data Sources", Chapter 7 in *Migration of Health Workers: WHO Code of Practice and the Global Economic Crisis*, WHO, Geneva.

4.2. Importance of foreign-trained doctors and nurses in OECD countries

Health workers trained abroad have generally contributed to the rise in the number and density of doctors and nurses in OECD countries since 2000 (see Figures 2.4 and 2.5 in Chapter 2), although all OECD countries are both destination countries and sending countries but to various extent.

There are important differences across OECD countries in the proportion of health workers trained abroad. In 2014 (or the most recent year available), the share of foreign-trained doctors ranged from less than 3% in Turkey, Poland, Estonia and the Czech Republic to more than 40% in Israel and New Zealand. In nearly all countries, the proportion of foreign-trained nurses is much lower than that of foreign-trained doctors. However, given that the overall number of nurses in most countries is greater than the number of doctors, the absolute number of foreign-trained nurses tends to be greater in most countries. While there are almost no foreign-trained nurses in countries such as Estonia, Poland and Slovenia, they make up nearly 25% of the nursing workforce in New Zealand, and between 15% and 20% in Australia and Switzerland (Tables 4.1 and 4.2).

Israel, New Zealand, Norway, Ireland and Australia have the highest share of foreign-trained doctors, with more than 30% of doctors trained abroad. Following these countries are the United Kingdom, Switzerland, the United States, Canada and Sweden, with rates between 24% and 30%. The very high proportion of foreign-trained doctors in Israel reflects not only the importance of immigration in this country, but also the fact that an increasing number of new licenses are issued to people born in Israel but trained abroad (about one-third in 2014). Similarly, in Norway, large numbers of Norwegians study medicine abroad (often with financial support from the State Educational Loan Fund), with the vast majority of them returning to practice in Norway.

In Nordic countries, the share of foreign-trained doctors varies from 6% in Denmark, to 20% in Finland, 24% in Sweden and 37% in Norway. Foreign-trained nurses still comprise less than 3% of the workforce in these first three countries, while they account for a greater share in Norway (9%).

In absolute numbers, the United States has by far the highest number of foreign-trained health workers, with more than 200 000 doctors trained abroad in 2013 and almost 250 000 nurses. Following the United States is the United Kingdom (with more than 48 000 foreign-trained doctors and 86 000 foreign-trained nurses in 2014), and Germany (with nearly 29 000 foreign doctors in 2014 and 70 000 foreign nurses in 2010, latest year available).

Since 2000, the number and proportion of foreign-trained doctors has increased in most OECD countries, although the share has levelled off in several countries in recent years. This has been the case in the United States and the United Kingdom, where the share has remained relatively stable and even fell slightly between 2006 and 2013-14, as the absolute number of doctors trained abroad coming into the country has increased more slowly than domestically-trained doctors.

Some countries have recorded a strong and steady increase in the number and share of foreign-trained doctors over the past decade. These include Sweden, Switzerland and France. In Sweden, the strong rise was driven mainly by foreign-trained doctors coming from Germany, Poland and Iraq. In Switzerland, the increase came mainly from neighbouring countries (Germany, Austria, Italy and France). In France, the rise was partly due to a fuller recognition of the qualifications of doctors who were already working in the country, but there have also been significant new inflows of doctors coming from new EU member states, notably Romania.

Recent trends in the migration patterns of foreign-trained nurses also vary across countries. There has been a strong rise in the immigration of foreign-trained nurses in Italy, primarily driven by the arrival of nurses trained in Romania, who accounted for over 40% of the annual registrations of nurses trained abroad in recent years. The movement of Romanian nurses to Italy preceded Romania's entry in the European Union in 2007. In other EU countries such as France and Belgium, the percentage of nurses trained abroad remains low, but their numbers have steadily increased. They have more than doubled in France between 2000 and 2014 and been multiplied by eight in Belgium. However, in some other countries (e.g., the Netherlands, Portugal and the United Kingdom), there has been a reduction in the number and proportion of foreign-trained nurses between 2006 and 2014 (or the most recent year available).

Table 4.1. Foreign-trained doctors working in 26 OECD countries, 2000, 2006 and 2012-14

Country of residence	2000				2006				2012-2014			
	Year	Total	Foreign-trained	% of total	Year	Total	Foreign-trained	% of total	Year	Total	Foreign-trained	% of total
Australia	2000	...	...	...	2005	...	...	25.0%	2013	82 498	25 153	30.5%
Austria	2000	25 611[e]	461	1.8%	2006	30 236	888	2.9%	2014	35 844	1 640	4.6%
Belgium	2000	44 380	1 934	4.4%	2006	49 695	2 636	5.3%	2014	59 070	6 732	11.4%
Canada	2000	64 462	13 701	21.3%	2006	70 870	15 237	21.5%	2013	90 205	21 225	23.5%
Chile	2000	...	...	...	2006	...	...	...	2014	36 013	5 489	15.2%
Czech Republic	2000	43 765	579	1.3%	2006	44 064	1 744	4.0%	2014	41 671	1 135	2.7%
Denmark	2000	15 551	681	4.4%	2006	18 403	1 145	6.2%	2012	20 250	1 127	5.6%
Estonia	2002	2 259	0	0.0%	2006	5 336	30	0.6%	2014	6 294	166	2.6%
Finland	2000	...	...	...	2005	...	...	...	2012	20 866	4 154	19.9%
France	2000	199 445	7 795	3.9%	2006	212 711	12 261	5.8%	2013	219 833	20 275	9.2%
Germany[1]	2000	267 965	9 971	3.7%	2006	284 427	14 703	5.2%	2013	326 945	28 901	8.8%
Hungary	2000	...	...	...	2006	37 908	2 917	7.7%	2013	32 668	2 470	7.6%
Ireland	2000	12 243[e]	1 359	11.1%	2006	15 512[e]	4 663	30.1%	2014	19 066	6 877	36.1%
Israel	2000	21 869	14 080	64.4%	2006	23 890	14 746	61.7%	2014	25 570	14 839	58.0%
Netherlands	2001	39 772	706	1.8%	2006	45 051	941	2.1%	2011	51 939	1 352	2.6%
New Zealand	2000	9 890	3 756	38.0%	2006	11 889	4 833	40.7%	2014	14 786	6 298	42.6%
Norway	2000	...	...	...	2008	18 557	5 996	32.3%	2014	22 659	8 447	37.3%
Poland	2000	...	...	...	2008	119 604	2 529	2.1%	2012	125 073	2 203	1.8%
Slovak Republic	2000	18 571[e]	130	0.7%	2004	17 375[e]	139	0.8%	2011	16 899	506	3.0%
Slovenia	2000	...	...	...	2006	...	...	...	2013	5 416	781	14.4%
Spain	2000	...	...	...	2006	...	...	...	2011	207 042	19 462	9.4%
Sweden	2000	27 502	3 827	13.9%	2006	32 802	6 321	19.3%	2012	38 144	9 283	24.3%
Switzerland	2000	25 272[e]	2 982	11.8%	2008	29 653	6 479	21.8%	2012	31 858	8 617	27.0%
Turkey	2000	85 242	55	0.1%	2006	104 475	240	0.2%	2013	133 775	261	0.2%
United Kingdom[2]	2000	...	...	...	2008	146 834	43 885	29.9%	2014	172 561	48 766	28.3%
United States[3]	2000	...	...	25.5%	2006	664 814	166 810	25.1%	2013	859 470	214 438	25.0%
OECD Total (26 countries)										**2 696 415**	**460 597**	**17.1%**

Note: Doctors whose place of training is unknown have been excluded from the calculation of the percentage of foreign-trained doctors (Netherlands, Slovak Republic, Slovenia and United Kingdom).

1. The data refer to foreign citizens (not necessarily foreign-trained).

2. Data cover England, Wales and Scotland (but not Northern Ireland).

3. The percentage in 2000 is calculated based on all doctors registered to practise. Data for 2006 and 2013 refer to doctors who are professionally active.

e: estimation.

Source: See Annex 4.A1.

StatLink http://dx.doi.org/10.1787/888933326261

Table 4.2. Foreign-trained nurses working in 25 OECD countries, 2000, 2006 and 2012-14

	2000				2006				2012-2014			
Country of residence	Year	Total	Foreign-trained	% of total	Year	Total	Foreign-trained	% of total	Year	Total	Foreign-trained	% of total
Australia	2000	...	...	...	2007	263 332	38 108	14.5%	2013	296 029	47 507	16.0%
Belgium	2000	130 560	679	0.5%	2006	150 817	1 290	0.9%	2014	186 278	5 411	2.9%
Canada	2000	232 566	14 187	6.1%	2006	326 170	21 445	6.6%	2013	375 768	28 330	7.5%
Chile	2000	...	...	...	2006	...	...	...	2014	34 674	702	2.0%
Denmark[1]	2000	49 694	889	1.8%	2006	51 840	818	1.6%	2012	55 037	724	1.3%
Estonia	2000	...	...	...	2006	10 264	...	...	2014	12 519	4	0.0%
Finland[2]	2000	...	...	0.2%	2005	...	...	0.3%	2012	72 471	1 293	1.8%
France	2000	404 564	7 016	1.7%	2006	493 503	11 712	2.4%	2014	622 052	17 692	2.8%
Germany[3]	2000	...	...	...	2006	...	...	...	2010	1 211 000	70 000	5.8%
Hungary	2000	...	...	...	2006	...	...	...	2013	53 323	650	1.2%
Ireland	2000	...	...	...	2004	60 819[e]	8 758	14.4%	2013	...	...	...
Israel	2000	39 064	7 277	18.6%	2006	43 481	6 077	14.0%	2014	45 982	4 528	9.8%
Italy	2000	304 159	1 825	0.6%	2006	358 746	15 108	4.2%	2014	424 813	20 072	4.7%
Netherlands	2001	169 580	1 495	0.9%	2006	186 990	2 149	1.1%	2011	198 694	1 358	0.7%
New Zealand	2002	33 027	4 860	14.7%	2008	39 247	8 931	22.8%	2014	45 572	11 170	24.5%
Norway	2000	...	...	...	2008	70 575	5 022	7.1%	2014	83 647	7 640	9.1%
Poland	2000	...	...	...	2008	268 015	5	0.0%	2012	278 496	7	0.0%
Portugal	2002	41 902	1 954	4.7%	2006	51 095	2 285	4.5%	2013	65 868	1 947	3.0%
Slovenia	2000	...	...	...	2006	...	...	...	2013	4 797	20	0.4%
Spain	2000	...	...	...	2006	...	...	...	2011	250 277	5 247	2.1%
Sweden	2000	88 302	2 358	2.7%	2006	98 905	2 789	2.8%	2012	106 176	2 882	2.7%
Switzerland	2000	...	...	...	2006	...	...	...	2012	61 609	11 536	18.7%
Turkey	2000	69 550	11	0.0%	2006	82 626	79	0.1%	2013	139 544	239	0.2%
United Kingdom[4]	2001	632 050[e]	50 564	8.0%	2006	659 470	88 609	13.4%	2014	683 625	86 668	12.7%
United States[5]	2000	...	...	...	2006	...	...	...	2012	4 104 854[e]	246 291[e]	6.0%
OECD Total (25 countries)										**9 413 105**	**571 918**	**6.1%**

Note: Nurses whose place of training is unknown are excluded from the calculation of the percentage of foreign-trained nurses (e.g. Switzerland).

1. The data only include professional nurses (and exclude associate professional nurses).

2. The data refer only to general nurses.

3. The data refer to citizens born abroad, not German by birth (except ethnic German repatriates) and to the highest degree in nursing acquired in a foreign country.

4. Different source in 2001 (Aiken et al., 2004).

5. Data refer to all nurses registered to practice.

e: estimation.

Source: See Annex 4.A1.

StatLink http://dx.doi.org/10.1787/888933326272

4.3. Changing composition of foreign-trained doctors and nurses in OECD countries

Foreign-trained health workers in OECD countries continue to come, in many cases, from other OECD countries (Table 4.3). This is the case in many English-speaking countries where a major source of migration is from other English-speaking countries. For example, more than 40% of migrant physicians in New Zealand were trained in the United Kingdom. In the United States, Canada and the United Kingdom are among the main countries of origin for foreign-trained doctors, although a greater number come from Mexico (and an even much greater number come from India, the Philippines and Pakistan). Migration patterns in the OECD are often linked to historical ties, the sharing of a common language and the reduction of other barriers to mobility, especially for Europeans moving within Europe.

Table 4.3. Main countries of origin of foreign-trained doctors in the United States, United Kingdom and New Zealand

United States (2013)		United Kingdom (2014)		New Zealand (2014)	
Total	**214 438**	**Total**	**48 766**	**Total**	**6 298**
OECD	50 856	OECD	10 225	OECD	4 144
Mexico	*10501*	*Ireland*	*1859*	*United Kingdom*	*2608*
Canada	*8444*	*Germany*	*1347*	*Australia*	*401*
United Kingdom	*4707*	*Greece*	*1162*	*United States*	*373*
India	47 271	India	16 833	South Africa	720
Philippines	11 973	Pakistan	5 275	India	468
Pakistan	11 779	Nigeria	2 189	Sri Lanka	138
Grenada	8 847	Egypt	1 718	Iraq	104
Dominica	8 072	South Africa	1 424	Pakistan	76
Dominican Rep.	6 302	Sri Lanka	1 354	China	75
Russia	5 925	Iraq	1 343	Fiji	68
China	5 442	Romania	848	Bangladesh	51
Egypt	4 366	Sudan	729	Egypt	51
Syria	3 852	Bangladesh	536	Russia	45

Note: Most physicians trained in Grenada, Dominica and the Dominican Republic are people with American nationality training abroad in preparation for return to practise in the United States (see Box 4.3).

Source: See Annex 4.A1.

StatLink http://dx.doi.org/10.1787/888933326280

India and the Philippines are by far the two most important countries of origin of foreign-trained doctors (India) and nurses (Philippines) working in OECD countries. This is not a new phenomenon as these two countries were already well ahead in 2000. The migration of doctors trained in India has traditionally been particularly strong in the United States, although the number of new registrations of Indian doctors in the United States has declined sharply in recent years (Figure 4.1). Still, the total number of doctors trained in India practising in the United States in 2013 reached more than 47 000. In the United Kingdom also, the annual inflow of doctors trained in India has come down in recent years, but the total number still exceeds by a wide margin those trained in any other countries (reaching nearly 17 000 in 2014). In both the United States and the United Kingdom, a large number of foreign-trained doctors have been trained in Pakistan (nearly 12 000 in the United States in 2013 and more than 5 000 in the United Kingdom in 2014).

Figure 4.1. Annual flow of doctors trained in India and Pakistan who migrated to the United States, 2002-13

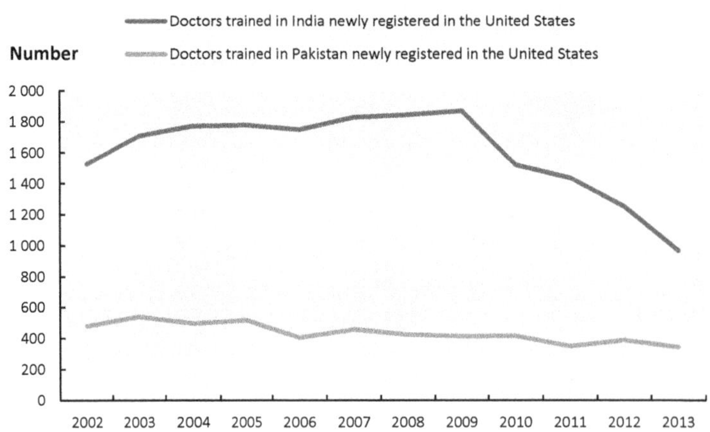

Source: American Medical Association, Physician Master Files.

StatLink http://dx.doi.org/10.1787/888933326297

During the 2000s, the Philippines has been the leading country of origin of migrant nurses in OECD countries. The United States was their main destination, reaching a peak of 10 000 Filipino nurses passing the examination to practise in that country in 2007. Following a decline in the demand for foreign nurses related to greater domestic training along with a greater retention and postponement of the retirement age of many nurses in the United States (Auerbach et al., 2014), the number of Filipino nurses who passed the exam has fallen sharply in recent years to reach only 1 000 in 2013. The United Kingdom and, to a lesser extent Ireland, have also recruited a significant number of nurses trained in the Philippines, mostly in the early 2000s, but the number has declined significantly in recent years (Figure 4.2).

Figure 4.2. Annual flow of nurses trained in the Philippines who migrated to the United States, the United Kingdom and Ireland, 2000-13

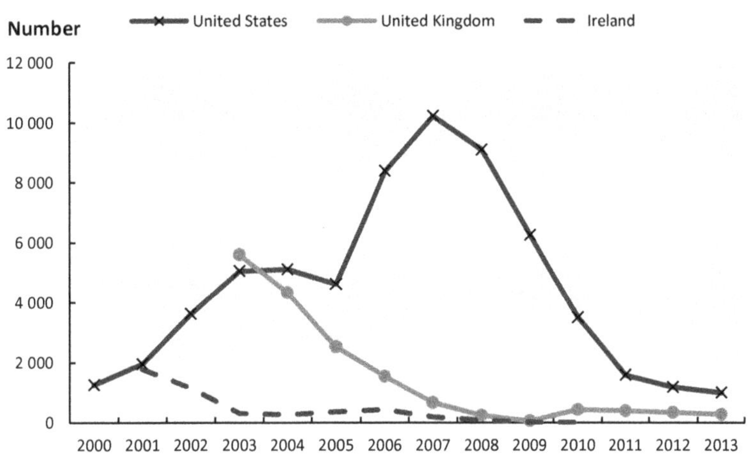

Note: In the United States, data refer to the number of trained nurses in the Philippines who passed the examination to be a registered nurse. In the United Kingdom and Ireland, data are for new registrations on professional registers. Between 2003 and 2008, data for the United Kingdom correspond to the administrative period ending March 31 of the year indicated. Data for Ireland are only available for the period 2001-10.

Source: National Council of State Boards of Nursing (NCSBN), NCLEX Examination Statistics (United States); Nursing and Midwifery Council (United Kingdom); Irish Nursing Board (Ireland).

StatLink http://dx.doi.org/10.1787/888933326303

Apart from English-speaking countries, other OECD countries have also experienced significant immigration of foreign-trained doctors and nurses. As already noted, in Italy, the number of nurses trained in Romania increased from less than 100 in 2000 to 11 000 in 2012, but the new annual inflow has decreased sharply in recent years. In France, Romania has become the second most important country of training of foreign-trained doctors (after Belgium), with a total number of around 3 500 Romanian-trained doctors having migrated by 2013, but the annual inflow appears to have started to decline (Figure 4.3).

In Spain, foreign-trained doctors come mainly from Latin America. Of the 3 200 new foreign-trained doctors registered in Spain in 2011, 500 were trained in Colombia. The Dominican Republic, Peru, Cuba and Venezuela were the next main countries of origin, with about 300 doctors each. Switzerland experienced a significant increase in the number of doctors trained in Germany in recent years, going up from 3 600 to 4 900 between 2008 and 2012.

Figure 4.3. Annual flow of doctors and nurses trained in Romania who migrated to France and Italy, 2000-13

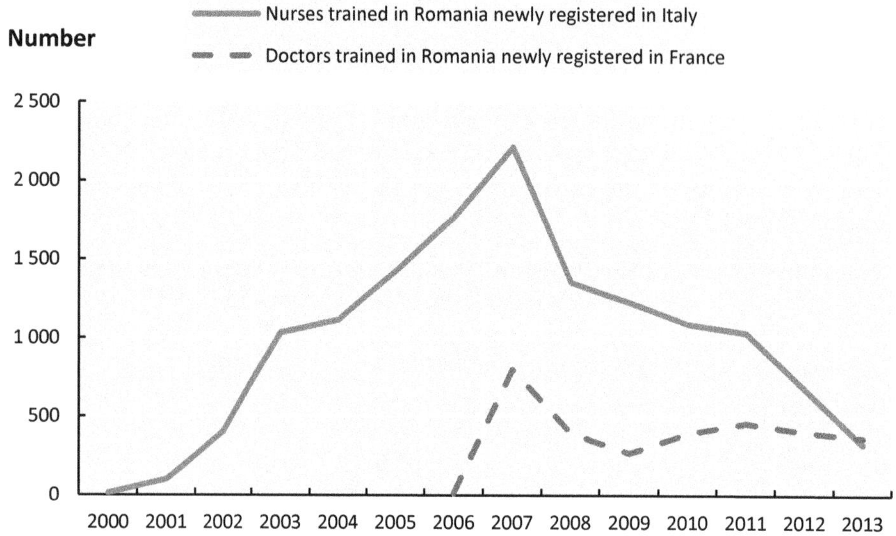

Source: Register of the College of Physicians (France) and Federazione nazionale dei Collegi Ipasvi (Italy).

StatLink http://dx.doi.org/10.1787/888933326310

4.4. Interactions between domestic education policies and international recruitment of doctors and nurses

Policies regarding the domestic education and training of doctors, nurses and other health professionals are, in most countries, the most important way of increasing the supply of health workers. Training enough health workers to reduce the need to recruit foreign-trained workers is one of the key principles of the WHO Global Code of Practice on the International Recruitment of Health Personnel (WHO, 2010). As shown in Chapter 3 of this publication, many OECD countries have increased substantially their medical and nursing education and training efforts since 2000 in response to concerns about current or future shortages. The increase in admission rates and graduation rates from medical and nursing education programmes, combined with the impact of the economic crisis in reducing at least temporarily the demand, has reduced the need to recruit foreign-trained doctors and nurses.

The United States provides a striking example of how a substantial increase in domestic training efforts for nurses may reduce the need to recruit foreign-trained nurses. Between 2001 and 2012, the number of domestically-trained nurses passing the certification exam more than doubled, rising from less than 70 000 in 2001 to nearly 150 000 in 2012 (Figure 4.4, right panel). This was accompanied by a sharp drop in the number of foreign-trained nurses who passed that exam, coming down from a peak of around 23 000 in 2007 to only about 5 000 in 2012. Up until now, the number of newly-registered doctors who got their initial degree in another country has remained more stable, at least up until 2012, but with the number of domestically-trained doctors continuing to go up, it can be expected that fewer foreign-trained doctors will become registered in the United States in the coming years (Figure 4.4, left panel).

Figure 4.4. Changes in the number of domestic graduates and inflow of foreign-trained health workers, United States, 2001-13

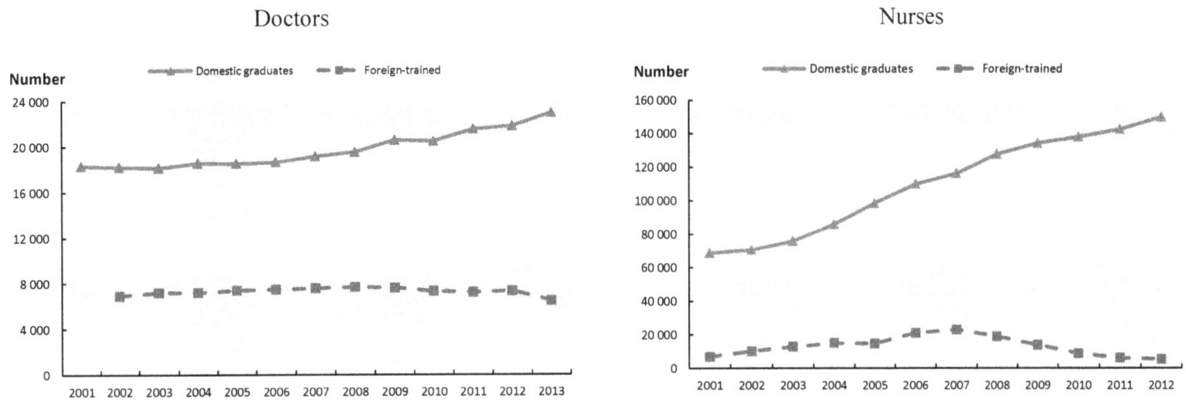

Source: The US Nursing Workforce: Trends in Supply and Education, Health Resources, Services Administration (HRSA), 2013; American Medical Associations, National Centre for Health Statistics.

StatLink http://dx.doi.org/10.1787/888933326324

In the United Kingdom, the steady rise in the number of domestic medical graduates since 2002 has also reduced the need to recruit abroad (Figure 4.5), although the annual inflow of foreign-trained doctors seems to have stabilised in recent years. But the countries of origin of foreign-trained doctors in the United Kingdom have changed considerably over the past decade, with a growing proportion of doctors trained in other EU countries. Regarding nurses, the inflow of foreign-trained nurses fell sharply between 2004 and 2009, but it has steadily gone up since then, driven mainly by the migration of nurses trained in other EU countries (e.g., Spain and Portugal), to meet growing demands for nurses that are not fully met by the growing supply of domestically-trained nurses. It is important to keep in mind that there are also large outflows of nurses trained in the United Kingdom, who are emigrating in other English-speaking countries such as Australia, Canada, New Zealand and the United States (Buchan and Seccombe, 2012).

Figure 4.5. Changes in the number of domestic graduates and inflow of foreign-trained health workers, United Kingdom, 2000-14 (or nearest year)

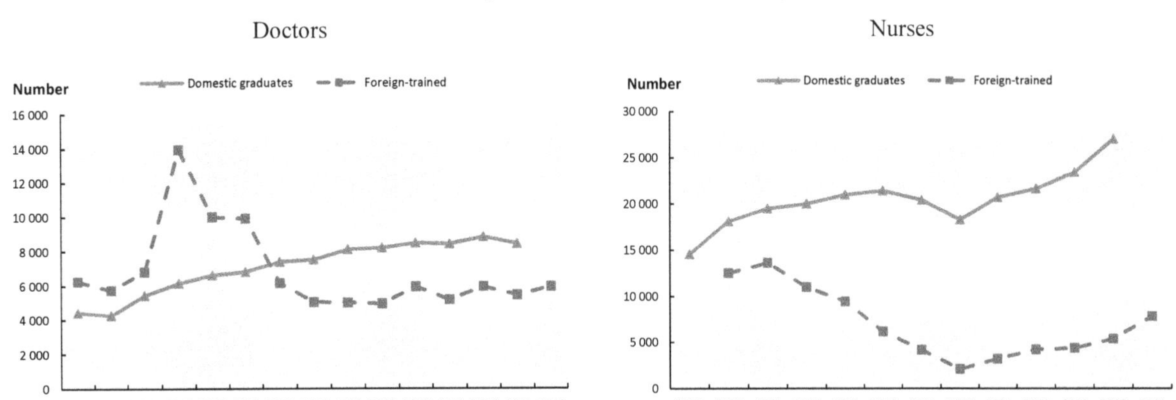

Note: Between 2005 and 2008, data on staff trained abroad correspond to the administrative period ending 31 March of the year indicated. Break in 2008 for the graduate series. Data from 2008 onwards are estimated.

Source: UK Graduate Output 1991/92 to 2012/13, Health and Social Care Information Centre. Nursing and Midwifery Council.

StatLink http://dx.doi.org/10.1787/888933326334

In Canada, the number of new domestic medical graduates and foreign-trained doctors are following similar upward trends since the early 2000s, contributing to the strong growth in the supply of physicians (Figure 4.6). The sharp increase in the number of domestically-trained nurses has been accompanied by stable inflows in foreign-trained nurses over the past decade. The fluctuations in the registration of nurses trained abroad during this period were driven mainly by variations in nurses coming from the Philippines.

Figure 4.6. Changes in the number of domestic graduates and inflow of foreign-trained health workers, Canada, 2000-13

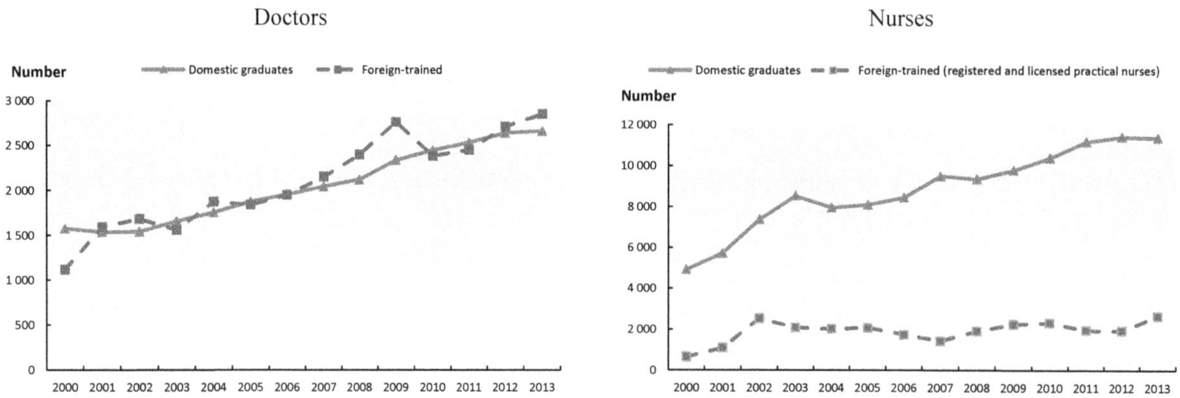

Note: The number of nursing graduates only includes those graduating from registered nurses (RN) programmes. In 2012, the total number of students graduating from a nursing programme was nearly 19 000 (including both Registered nurses and Licensed practical nurses).

Source: CIHI, Scotts Medical Database (SMDB); CNA and CASN, CIHI, Nursing Database.

StatLink http://dx.doi.org/10.1787/888933326349

In New Zealand, the immigration of foreign-trained doctors has exceeded by far the number of domestic graduates in the country in all years since 2000 (Figure 4.7). For nurses, the increase in the number of domestic graduates, particularly since 2009, has led to a situation where domestic graduates now exceed by a significant margin the number of foreign-trained nurses. In recent years, nurses migrating to New Zealand have come mainly from the Philippines and India.

Figure 4.7. Changes in the number of domestic graduates and inflow of foreign-trained health workers, New Zealand, 2000-14

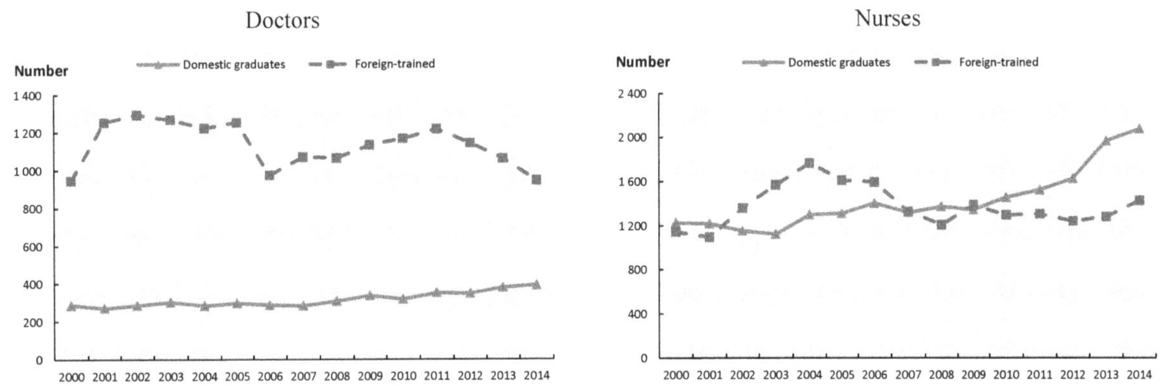

Source: Medical Council of New Zealand (MCNZ), Nursing Council of New Zealand.

StatLink http://dx.doi.org/10.1787/888933326354

Figure 4.8. Changes in the number of domestic graduates and foreign-trained health workers, the Netherlands, 2000-13 (or nearest year)

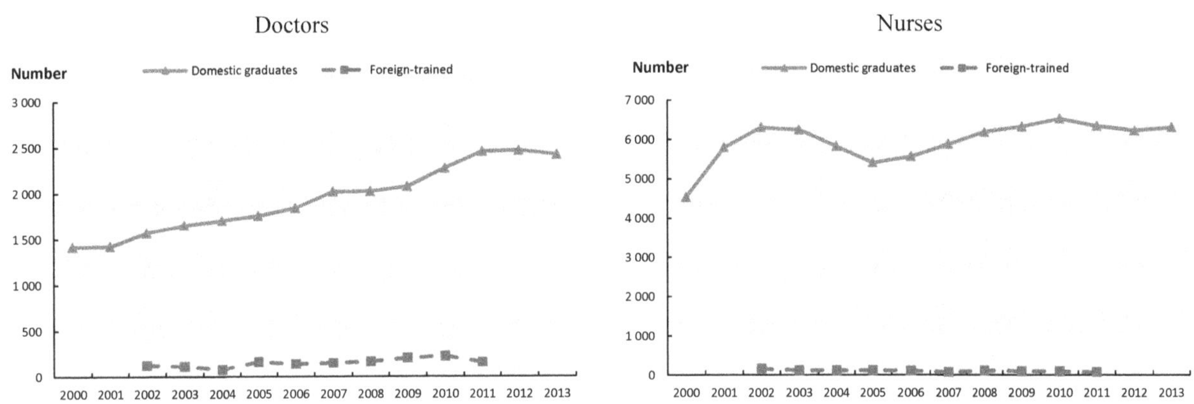

Source: BIG Register; Statistics Netherlands, Statistics of Education.

StatLink http://dx.doi.org/10.1787/888933326363

In the Netherlands, the number of new domestic medical graduates has steadily increased since 2002, while the annual inflow of foreign-trained doctors has remained relatively marginal. The number of new graduates from nursing programmes has been more stable (following a temporary drop in the mid-2000s), and the inflow of foreign-trained nurses has remained very low (Figure 4.8).

Annex 4.A2 shows similar figures comparing inflows from domestically-trained and foreign-trained doctors and nurses for several other countries.

As noted above, among all the foreign-trained doctors and nurses who are working in OECD countries, a certain number might actually be national citizens who got their degree in another country and have come back to complete their training and work in their home country. This phenomenon can be expected to become more common given the growing internationalisation of higher-level education. The growing opportunities for students to get their medical or nursing education in another country might help to increase the total number of new medical and nursing graduates, but some of these students may face bottlenecks to complete their training and to practice if the number of post-graduate training places in medicine (internship and residency) in the country where they have studied or in their home country does not grow at the same pace or if there is not enough new positions to absorb all the new graduates (in the case of nursing) (Box 4.3).

Box 4.3. Will all the new international medical graduates be able to get post-graduate training places to complete their training and practice?

The internationalisation of medical education has grown very rapidly in recent years, with many universities in different countries competing to attract foreign students to increase their size and revenues. The growing number of students pursuing their medical education in another country often have the intention of coming back to their home countries to pursue their post-graduate training and to work. For example, in 2013, 43% of the 7 100 doctors trained abroad who registered with the American Medical Association were in fact American citizens who came back after acquiring their first medical degree, in most cases from universities in Caribbean countries that specialise in the training of foreign students (Dominica, Grenada, Saint Martin). In the European Union, student mobility has been encouraged by the Directive on the recognition of professional qualifications (Directive 2005/36/EC, which was amended in 2013 by Directive 2013/55/EU). Several universities in Central and Eastern European countries (Czech Republic, Poland, Slovak Republic, Hungary, Romania, and Bulgaria) have set up courses in English, French and German to attract students from other EU and non-EU countries.

One issue that the rising number of international medical students has already started to pose is whether there will be enough post-graduate training places to allow them to complete their studies either in the country where they have obtained their first medical degree or in their home country (particularly if they are required to do these internships/residencies in their home country if they want to be fully recognised afterwards as is the case in the United States and Canada for example). The number of places in post-graduate training programmes is generally regulated in most countries and limited by the capacity to offer proper training places in hospital or in other settings and by the projected needs for doctors. If the number of internships or residency positions does not grow at the same pace as the number of medical graduates, there is a real risk that many medical graduates will not have the opportunity to complete their training and work as doctors, resulting in a huge loss of several years of education and money, and this problem is likely to fall first and foremost on international medical graduates. In the United States and Canada, there are already strong pressures to loosen up this bottleneck to allow a greater number of international medical students (notably American and Canadian students coming back) to complete their medical training, but the room to expand the number of places in these post-graduate training programmes is not unlimited and involves significant public cost.

4.5. Emigration patterns from some European countries following EU enlargement and the economic crisis

The accession of ten new member states to the European Union in 2004, two more in 2007 and one more in 2013, had a significant effect on the emigration of health workers from some of these countries, although this effect has been temporary in some cases and reduced in recent years.

The migration of health workers within the European Union has been facilitated by the recognition of professional qualifications under Directive 2005/36/EC which came into effect in October 2007. This Directive covers a set of professions for which minimum training conditions have been harmonised, including the medical and nursing professions. It allows for the automatic recognition of qualifications obtained after a specific reference date. Qualifications awarded before that date may be recognised on the basis of acquired rights. People with the required qualifications must be able to demonstrate sufficient professional experience (over a certain period of time). In November 2013, the European Parliament adopted Directive 2013/55/EU, amending Directive 2005/36/EC. This new Directive called for the introduction of a

European Professional Card, taking the form of an electronic certificate duly validated by both the source and destination countries, to further facilitate mobility. This Professional Card was introduced in January 2016, initially covering five professions of which three are in the health sector (general care nurses, pharmacists and physiotherapists). It may be extended to other professions in the future. The new 2013 Directive also sought to clarify the language requirements relating to the recognition of qualifications, reaffirming that, in principle, the verification of language skills should follow a procedure different from that involved in the recognition of qualifications.

Following the EU enlargement and the implementation of this Directive on the recognition of professional qualifications, there has been, as expected, a growing mobility of doctors and nurses across EU countries. Germany has been a particularly important destination country for many European physicians, particularly those in Central and Eastern Europe (Figure 4.9). The emigration of Polish doctors to Germany has stabilised, after an initial surge following the entry of Poland in the European Union in 2004. On the other hand, the emigration of Hungarian doctors to Germany has steadily risen since its entry into the European Union. In the case of Romania, the combined effect of the economic crisis and accession to the European Union in 2007 has led to a massive increase in the emigration of Romanian doctors to Germany, which possibly reached a peak in 2012. The migration of Greek doctors to Germany has also increased steadily since the early 2000s, and accelerated following the economic crisis in 2008.

Figure 4.9. Flow of foreign doctors in Germany, 2000-13

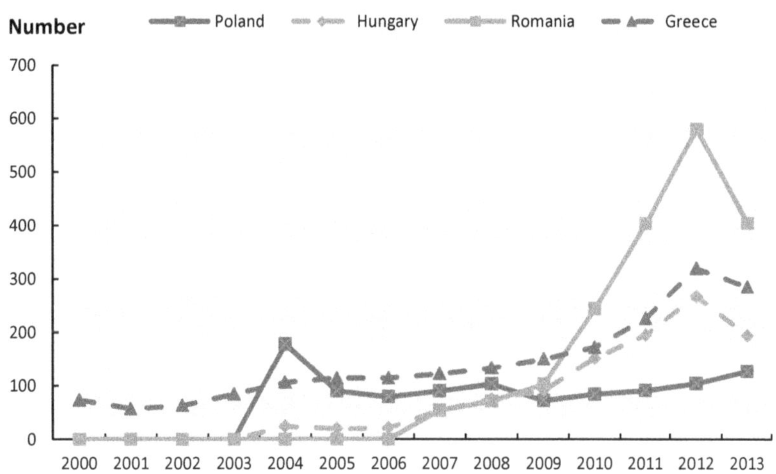

Note: Data refer to foreign doctors.

Source: German Medical Association.

StatLink http://dx.doi.org/10.1787/888933326371

In the United Kingdom, nurses coming from European countries hit hard by the economic crisis also increased sharply in recent years, notably from Spain and Portugal (Figure 4.10). The annual inflow of nurses coming from Poland reached a peak following the entry of Poland in the European Union in 2004, but has steadily decreased since then.

Figure 4.10. Trends in nurses trained abroad, United Kingdom, 2007-13

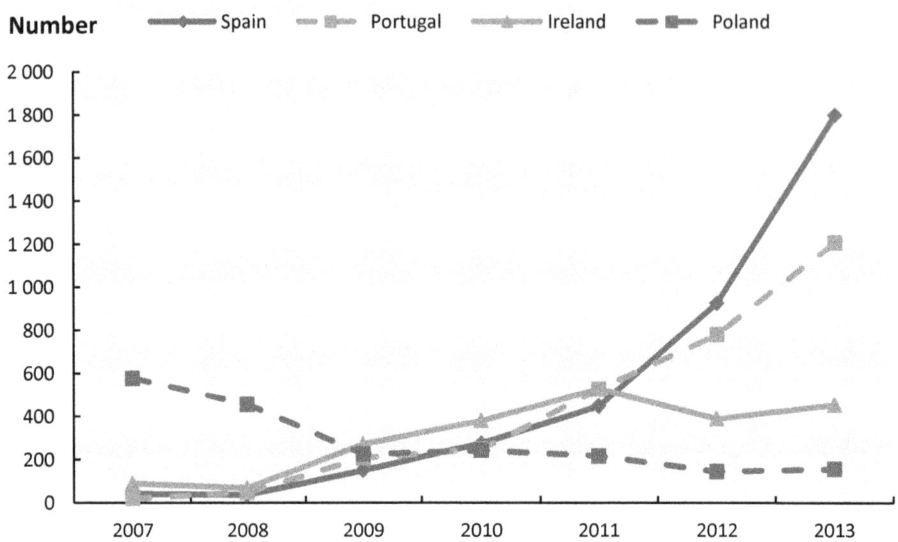

Note: Between 2005 and 2008, data on staff trained abroad correspond to the administrative period ending 31 March of the year indicated. Only data on nurses trained in Poland are available in 2005 and 2006.

Source: Nursing and Midwifery Council.

StatLink http://dx.doi.org/10.1787/888933326383

4.6. Recent policies to reduce the emigration of doctors and nurses in Central and Eastern European countries

The emigration of a large number of doctors and nurses from several Central and Eastern European countries to Western Europe countries following their accession to the European Union has raised serious concerns about increased shortages of health workers in many of these countries, particularly in rural areas that were already in short supply of doctors, or in certain specialties (e.g., anaesthesiologists, surgeons, emergency physicians, general practitioners). In Romania, the emigration of doctors and nurses has had a particularly strong effect on smaller hospitals, often located in more remote areas and which have more difficulties in recruiting and retaining staff (Buchan et al., 2014).

To reduce these losses of skilled health workers, several Central and Eastern European countries have introduced various measures in recent years to increase retention rates and even in some cases to encourage the return of those who have emigrated. Such measures have often come in the wake of a sudden increase in intentions to migrate and, in some countries, growing discontent among health workers about their pay and working conditions. In general, these retention measures have targeted doctors more than nurses.

In the Slovak Republic, a number of measures have been adopted to encourage doctors to stay in the country. With EU support, EUR 250 million has been earmarked for modernising health care infrastructures, recognising that inadequate facilities and equipment were one of the factors pushing doctors to leave. A programme of bursaries subsidised by the European Social Fund was also launched in 2008 for doctors pursuing specialisation studies, and this programme (called the "Operational Health Programme") was extended in 2009 to cover nurses and midwives. Recipients of these bursaries are expected to work in a predetermined region or health institution within the Slovak

Republic for a length of time equivalent to that of the duration of their bursary. The bursary must be repaid if the beneficiary does not fulfil this commitment. In 2012, 481 doctors and 864 nurses and midwives benefitted from this programme, funded by a budget of EUR 9.3 million (Ministry of Health of the Slovak Republic, 2011). Pay rates have also been increased substantially in response to protests by doctors, nurses and other health workers. This pay increase was being phased in between January 2012 and January 2015. In 2012 and 2013, the average salary for doctors rose by 26.5% (compared to 7.5% in the two previous years), and the average salary for nurses went up by 19% (compared to 5.5% in the previous two years).

In Hungary, a bursaries programme was also launched in 2011 for doctors pursuing their specialisation, also based on a requirement of a length of service in Hungary equivalent to the duration of the bursary. The bursary, which was initially set at around EUR 300 per month, increased significantly the salaries of many doctors in training. Since its introduction, around 600 out of the 800 to 900 doctors pursuing their specialisation have benefitted from this bursary programme. A staged increase of 20% in the salaries of doctors and nurses already working in the system was also introduced in 2012, phased over a three-year period. To finance these measures, the government introduced a *Public Health Product Tax* in 2011, imposed on foods and beverages deemed harmful to health.

In the Czech Republic, several thousand hospital doctors offered their resignations and threatened to leave the country in 2011. Following this protest, a memorandum of understanding was concluded with the Health Ministry. Doctors working in public institutions have seen their monthly salary rise by over 20% (from around EUR 1 800 in 2010 to about EUR 2 200 in 2012). This increase also benefited nurses, but to a lesser extent. The measures planned for increasing the retention of nursing staff focussed instead on improving their working conditions.

In Romania, the austerity measures imposed in 2010 included a 25% salary cut in the public sector and a freeze on hiring. These measures had a particularly strong impact on doctors undergoing specialisation. In order to curb their emigration, their salaries were gradually restored in 2011 and 2012 to their levels prior to the budget cuts. Preventing the departure of these doctors has remained a priority since then. In the autumn of 2013, a decree offered a bursary of EUR 150 a month, tax-free, to support doctors pursuing their specialisation in public institutions, if their gross monthly salary was less than EUR 670.

In Bulgaria, several initiatives co-financed by the European Structural Funds have provided financial support for doctors in specialisation, although these measures have been of modest scope and limited duration. A key problem is the lack of post-graduate training places financed publicly. Between 2009 and 2012, public funding for the training of doctors and nurses fell by 30% (Dussault and Buchan, 2014), and doctors have left the country in growing numbers.

It is difficult to measure precisely the impact of these retention measures on health worker migration patterns. In some cases, the number of applications for the recognition of professional qualifications (which is an indicator of the intention to emigrate) has dropped following the introduction of various financial incentives and other initiatives to improve working conditions. This is the case, for example, with doctors in Hungary and in Romania. The effects have been less visible for nurses.

4.7. Recent developments of bilateral or multilateral agreements on training and recruitment of health workers

In recent years, several OECD countries have implemented bilateral programmes or agreements for the international recruitment of health personnel with certain countries. None of the agreements reviewed here are designed specifically to implement the WHO Global Code of Practice, and some indeed preceded its adoption. However, by defining clearly the procedures and conditions governing any international recruitment, by targeting recruitment from countries or regions that do not have a shortage of health workers, and/or by encouraging professional integration and recognition of qualifications for health personnel, these programmes tend to promote a more ethical recruitment. These bilateral agreements are designed to provide mutual benefits to both countries of origin and countries of destination, as well as for the migrants themselves.

Germany concluded a bilateral agreement with Vietnam in 2012, covering pilot projects for the training and recruitment of geriatric nurses in Vietnam. This country was identified on the basis of its strategy of training nurses for the global market. The project was commissioned by the German Federal Ministry of Economics and Technology (BMWi) and is being implemented by the German co-operation agency (GIS) in collaboration with the Vietnamese Ministry of Labour, Invalids and Social Affairs. Some 100 Vietnamese nursing graduates were selected initially to take six months of training in the German language and culture. Participants then travelled to Germany at the end of 2013 to begin two years of professional training, accompanied by a programme of integration and language courses. This pilot project seeks to establish the basis for the future recruitment of skilled foreign personnel to provide care in Germany. At the same time, a project for recruiting nurses in China was launched by the German caregiving employers' association. Conditions for participation in this programme are a bachelor's degree, one year of professional experience, and eight months of language and cultural training. While awaiting recognition of their credentials, Chinese nurses work as nursing assistants. Germany expected to receive 150 Chinese nurses via this route in 2014.

The German authorities have also sought to ensure that, consistent with the principles of the WHO Code of Practice, its international recruitment activities would not come at the expense of the countries of origin. During the July 2013 review of the list of professions in short supply in Germany, the government prohibited the recruitment of health workers in the 57 countries that WHO identified in 2006 as facing a critical shortage. This decision was subsequently reconsidered, as it not only banned active recruitment by employers or private agencies but also prevented health workers from these countries to seek employment in Germany on their own initiative (so-called "passive recruitment"). This provision was finally removed in the revision of the employment ordinance in October 2013, which now only prohibits active recruitment and the private placement of health workers from these 57 countries.

In Finland, at least two international recruitment experiments are worth noting: the *DOKTOR* project (promoting work-based immigration of doctors), conducted by the University of Eastern Finland between 2008 and 2011, and the *Mediko* programme (promoting the recruitment of foreign health and social care professionals to Finland) also launched in 2008 and still in place. These two initiatives received funding from the European Social Funds as well as the local, regional and national public authorities. The *DOKTOR* project focused on recruiting doctors in the north-western part of the Russian Federation. These doctors worked first as assistants while following a training programme that included Finnish language courses and receiving professional and social integration help. They then took the examination required by the national health authority (Valvira) for practising medicine in Finland. Initially co-ordinated by the municipality of Kotka, the *Mediko* project was then expanded to cover all of Finland. Since its creation, *Mediko* has provided counselling to some 80 doctors, mainly Russian, wishing to practise in Finland. *Mediko* has also started to recruit nurses in Spain. Following an exploratory visit in 2012, 2 000 Spanish nurses expressed an interest in moving to Finland. Finnish language courses have been organised in various Spanish cities, and since 2012, nearly 150 people have been recruited via this route. Intensive language courses prior to departure are planned to bolster the motivation to move for longer-term recruitment. *Mediko* also promotes co-operation between Finnish training institutions and Spanish, Russian and Estonian institutions.

These international recruitment practices, conducted within the framework of co-operation agreements, might expand in the future, if they prove to be successful and of mutual benefits. Some of the key stakeholders involved in these initiatives are counting on the idea that once a chain of recruitment has started, it is likely to open up opportunities for a growing number of potential immigrants.

4.8. Conclusions

Foreign-trained doctors and nurses represent a significant share of doctors and nurses working in OECD countries. This share has increased in most OECD countries between 2000 and 2012-14, with the exception of the United Kingdom and the United States where the share of foreign-trained doctors decreased at least slightly since around 2006 due mainly to a rise in the number of domestic graduates from medical education programmes. To a certain extent, the rise in the number and share of foreign-trained doctors and nurses reflects the overall increase in immigration in OECD countries, notably of highly-skilled workers. A large proportion of these doctors and nurses (between one-fourth and one-third in 2010/11) were born in other OECD countries. Two Asian countries are also important places of origin – India for doctors and the Philippines for nurses – although their annual migration to OECD countries has decreased in recent years.

The increase in the number of immigrant health workers occurred in a context where many OECD countries have increased their efforts to train more doctors and nurses since 2000, and where the economic crisis of 2008 has at least temporarily reduced the demand for health workers in some countries. In most countries, the main source of new doctors and nurses in recent years has come from the growing number of domestic graduates in medicine and nursing.

In Europe, the combined effect of accession to the European Union (which have reduced barriers to mobility) and austerity measures following the economic crisis has led to substantial waves of emigration of doctors and nurses from Central and Eastern European countries to Western European countries (notably Germany) over the past decade, although in some cases the emigration outflows have come down after an initial surge (e.g., in the case of Poland). To improve health workforce retention and access to care, several Central and Eastern European countries have adopted measures to increase the pay rates of doctors and nurses and improve their working conditions, despite the fact that they were facing tight budget constraints.

By adopting the Global Code of Practice on the International Recruitment of Health Personnel in 2010, all countries have committed to improving their health workforce planning and to responding to their future needs without relying unduly on the training efforts of other countries, notably those already suffering from critical workforce shortages. The goal must not necessarily be to achieve self-sufficiency, but to avoid relying too much on other countries to fill domestic needs.

Beyond adjusting their education and training policies to meet future needs for doctors and nurses, OECD countries may also adopt a series of measures to improve the use of existing human resources and to increase retention rates, notably for nurses by improving their working conditions.

To address shortages and reduce emigration, countries that are losing a significant number of their skilled health workers may also need to do more to retain them, by improving their working conditions and pay rates. These measures will require good governance of the health system and long-term financial commitment, which in many cases may require the support of the international community.

Several bilateral or multilateral agreements have been reached in recent years to promote mutually beneficial co-operation and co-ordination in international recruitment of health personnel, under the broad principles proposed in the WHO Global Code. Up until now, most of these bilateral or multilateral agreements have involved a fairly limited number of doctors and/or nurses. If these agreements provide benefits for origin and destination countries, one might expect that their number and size will continue to grow in the years ahead.

Note

1. The authors are thankful to Irene Glinos (from the European Observatory on Health Systems and Policies) for providing useful inputs for the section on policies to promote the retention of doctors and nurses in Central and Eastern European countries and to Frédéric Daniel (OECD) for statistical assistance. A longer version of this chapter, presenting also information on foreign-born health workers working in OECD countries based on population census around 2010/11, was published in the *International Migration Outlook 2015* (Chapter 3), although the present chapter contains new information on health policies designed to reduce emigration rates. The preparation of this chapter has benefited from funding support from the World Health Organization and the Swiss Government. The content of this chapter is the sole responsibility of the OECD and can in no way be taken to reflect the views of the World Health Organization or any national government.

References

Aiken, L.H. and R. Cheung (2008), "Nurse Workforce Challenges in the United States: Implication for Policy", *OECD Health Working Papers No. 35*, OECD Publishing, Paris, http://dx.doi.org/10.1787/236153608331.

Aiken, L.H. et al. (2004), "Trends in International Nurse Migration", *Health Affairs*, Vol. 23, No. 3, pp. 69-77.

Auerbach, D.I., P.I. Buerhaus and O. Staiger (2014), "Registered Nurses Are Delaying Retirement, A Shift that Has Contributed to Recent Growth in the Nurse Workforce", *Health Affairs*, July.

Buchan, J. and I. Seccombe (2012), *Overstretched, Under-resourced: The UK Nursing Labour Market Review 2012*, Royal College of Nursing.

Buchan, J. et al. (2014), *Health Professional Mobility in a Changing Europe. New Dynamics, Mobile Individuals and Diverse Responses*, WHO-Europe.

Dumont, J.C., G. Lafortune and P. Zurn (2014), "Monitoring Trends in International Migration of Health Personnel: A Critical Review of Existing Data sources", Chapter 7 in *Migration of Health Workers: WHO Code of Practice and the Global Economic Crisis*, WHO, Geneva.

Dussault, G. and J. Buchan (2014), "The Economic Crisis in the EU: Impact on Health Workforce Mobility", *Health Professional Mobility in a Changing Europe. New Dynamics, Mobile Individuals and Diverse Responses*, WHO-Europe.

GMC – General Medical Council (2012), *The State of Medical Education and Practice in the UK*, General Medical Council.

Haklai, Z. et al. (2013), "Female Physicians: Trends and Likely Impacts on Healthcare in Israel", *Israel Journal of Health Policy Research*, Vol. 2, No. 37.

Ministry of Health of the Slovak Republic (2011), "For Action 2.2 of the Operational Programme Education 2012", European Programmes and Projects Directorate, Newsletter.

OECD (2015a), *OECD Health Statistics 2015*, OECD Publishing, Paris, http://www.oecd.org/els/health-systems/health-data.htm.

OECD (2015b), "Changing Patterns in the International Migration of Doctors and Nurses in OECD Countries", Chapter 3 in *International Migration Outlook 2015*, OECD, Paris, http://dx.doi.org/10.1787/migr_outlook-2015-6-en.

OECD (2008), *The Looming Crisis in the Health Workforce: How Can OECD Countries Respond?*, OECD Publishing, Paris, http://dx.doi.org/10.1787/9789264050440-en.

OECD (2007), "Immigrant Health Workers in OECD Countries in the Broader Context of Highly Skilled Migration", *International Migration Outlook,* OECD Publishing, Paris, http://dx.doi.org/10.1787/migr_outlook-2007-en.

WHO (2014), *Migration of Health Workers: WHO Code of Practice and the Global Economic Crisis*, Geneva.

WHO (2010), *WHO Global Code of Practice on the International Recruitment of Health Personnel,* Geneva.

Annex 4.A1
Data sources on foreign-trained doctors and nurses

Table 4.A1.1. Data sources on foreign-trained doctors

	Source	Comment
Australia	Australian Institute of Health and Welfare (AIHW).	Professionally active doctors, includes resident doctors.
Austria	Austrian Medical Chamber.	Practising doctors, includes resident doctors.
Belgium	Federal Public Service - Public Health, Database of health work professionals, (INAMI - RIZIV).	Includes health work professionals with a license to practice their profession.
Canada	Canadian Institute for Health Information, Scotts Medical Database (SMDB).	Professionally active doctors, includes resident doctors, but excludes doctors in the military and doctors who requested that their information not be published.
Chile	Health Superintendence - National Registry of Individual Health Providers.	All licensed doctors, includes resident doctors.
Czech Rep.	Czech Medical Chamber.	All licensed doctors, includes resident doctors.
Denmark	Statens Serum Institut, Population Register.	Practising doctors, includes resident doctors.
Estonia	Health Board, Register of Health Professionals.	All licensed doctors.
Finland	National Supervisory Authority for Welfare and Health (Valvira), Central Register of Health Care Professionals.	Licensed doctors, including resident doctors, but only includes doctors under the age of 64 and excludes specialists.
France	Direction de la Recherche, des études, de l'évaluation et des statistiques (DRESS) based on Adeli until 2010 and RPPS from 2011.	Professionally active doctors, does not include resident doctors.
Germany	German Medical Association.	Practising doctors, includes resident doctors. Data based on nationality (not place of training).
Hungary	Office of Health Authorisation and Administrative Procedures, Operational Registry.	Professionally active doctors, does not include resident doctors. Includes doctors who have a valid registration in the Operational Registry, which is the condition for unsupervised healthcare activity.
Ireland	Medical Council of Ireland.	Data refer to all licensed doctors. Includes doctors working outside Ireland.
Israel	Health Information Division, Ministry of Health, Physician License Registry.	All licensed doctors, includes resident doctors. Possible delay in removing inactive doctors.
Netherlands	CIBG, Beroepen in de Gezondheidszorg (BIG).	Professionally active doctors, includes resident doctors. Data on cross-border doctors working in the Netherlands are likely to be incomplete.
New Zealand	Medical Council of New Zealand, Medical Register.	Practising doctors, includes resident doctors, only includes permanent registrations.
Norway	Statistics Norway. Statistics on health-care personnel.	Professionally active doctors, includes interns and residents, although some of the doctors may be working in other occupations.
Poland	Polish Supreme Chamber of Physicians and Dentists, Central Register of Physicians and Dentists of the Republic of Poland.	Practising doctors, does not include resident doctors, possible delay in updating the register.
Slovak Rep.	National administrative register of healthcare professionals.	Practising doctors, includes resident doctors, about 60% of the total number of doctors are covered.
Slovenia	National Institute of Public Health Slovenia, National Healthcare Providers Database.	Practising doctors, includes resident doctors.
Spain	Regional Councils of Physicians, National Institute of Statistics.	Licensed doctors, for some regions, only data on nationality or country of birth are available.
Sweden	National Board of Health and Welfare, NPS-register.	Practising doctors, does not include resident doctors.
Switzerland	Fédération des médecins suisses (FMH).	Professionally active doctors, does not include resident doctors.
Turkey	General Directorate for Health Information Systems.	Professionally active doctors, include resident doctors.
United Kingdom	ISD (Scotland), HSCIC (England) and GMS Census (Wales).	Practising doctors, includes resident doctors and only doctors active in the public sector. Does not include data on Northern Ireland.
United States	Association of American Medical Colleges (AAMC) - GME Track.	Data reflect first-year residents entering ACGME-accredited residency programmes.

Table 4.A1.2. Data sources on foreign-trained nurses

	Source	Comment
Australia	Australian Institute of Health and Welfare (AIHW).	Professionally active nurses.
Belgium	Federal Public Service - Public Health, Database of health work professionals, (INAMI - RIZIV).	Licensed nurses.
Canada	Canadian Institute for Health Information, Health Workforce Database.	Professionally active nurses.
Chile	Health Superintendence - National Registry of Individual Health Providers.	Licensed nurses, only includes professional nurses (excludes lower-level nurses).
Denmark	Statens Serum Institut, Population Register.	Practising nurses, only includes professional nurses (excludes lower-level nurses).
Estonia	Health Board, Register of Health Professionals.	Licensed nurses.
Finland	National Supervisory Authority for Welfare and Health (Valvira), Central Register of Health Care Professionals.	Professionally active nurses, includes nurses under age 64.
France	Direction de la Recherche, des études, de l'évaluation et des statistiques (DRESS), Répertoire Adeli des professions de santé.	Professionally active nurses.
Germany	Federal Statistical Office in cooperation with the Federal Statistical Offices of the Länder, Statistics for the Federal Recognition Act (2012).	Practising nurses, includes geriatric nurses and midwives.
Hungary	Office of Health Authorisation and Administrative Procedures, Operational Registry.	Nurses with a valid registration in the Operational Registry (a condition for unsupervised practice).
Ireland	Irish Nursing Board, An Board Altranais	Only data on new registrations are available, only includes general nurses.
Israel	Health Information Division, Ministry of Health, Nurse License Registry.	Only includes nurses under age of 65. Includes nurses living abroad or working in another sector (these accounted for about 5% of all nurses on the register in 2008).
Italy	Federazione nazionale dei Collegi Ipasvi.	Data refer to nurses entitled to practice. Includes nurses registered in Italy but practising abroad.
Netherlands	CIBG, Beroepen in de Gezondheidszorg (BIG).	Professionally active nurses, data on cross-border nurses working in the Netherlands are likely to be incomplete.
New Zealand	Nursing Council of New Zealand, New Zealand Workforce Survey Data.	Practising nurses, includes professional nurses.
Norway	Statistics Norway; Statistics on health-care personnel. Administrative registers.	Professionally active nurses, although some of the nurses may be working in other occupations.
Poland	Main Chamber of Nurses and Midwifes, Central Register of Nurses and Midwifes.	Licensed nurses.
Portugal	Ordem dos Enfermeiros, Gestão de Membros da Ordem dos Enfermeiros.	Professionally active nurses.
Slovenia	National Institute of Public Health Slovenia, National Healthcare Providers Database.	Practising nurses, only includes professional nurses (excludes lower-level nurses).
Spain	Regional Councils of Nurses, National Institute of Statistics.	Licensed nurses, for some regions, only data on nationality or country of birth are available.
Sweden	National Board of Health and Welfare, NPS-register.	Practising nurses.
Switzerland	FSO Swiss Federal Statistical Office, Administrative Hospital Statistics.	Practising nurses, only includes nurses working in hospital (these data are not representative of the nursing population as a whole).
Turkey	General Directorate for Health Information Systems.	Professionally active nurses.
United Kingdom	Nursing and Midwifery Council – Wiser database.	Practising nurses.
United States	2013 National Workforce Survey of Registered Nurses, National Council of State Boards of Nursing.	Professionally active nurses, includes registered nurses, nurses trained in Guam, Puerto Rico, Virgin Islands or any other unspecified U.S. territory are not included.

Annex 4.A2
Trends in the number of domestic medical and nursing graduates and inflow of foreign-trained doctors and nurses in some OECD countries

Figure 4.A2.1. Changes in the number of domestic medical and nursing graduates and inflow of foreign-trained doctors and nurses, selected OECD countries, 2000-14 (or nearest year)

Doctors, Denmark, 2000-14

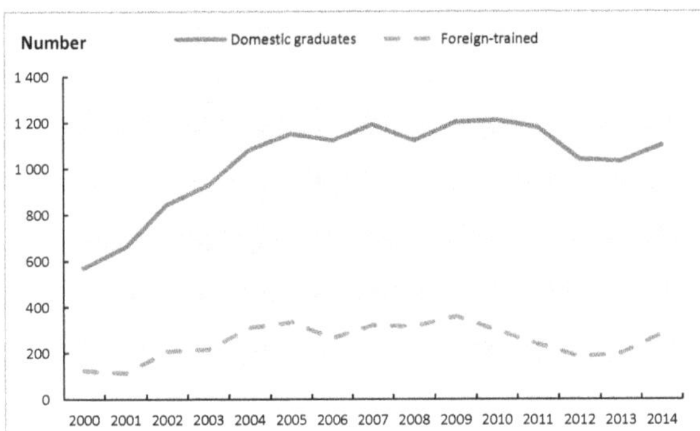

Source: National Board of Health and Statens Serum Institut, Population Register.

Nurses, Denmark, 2000-14

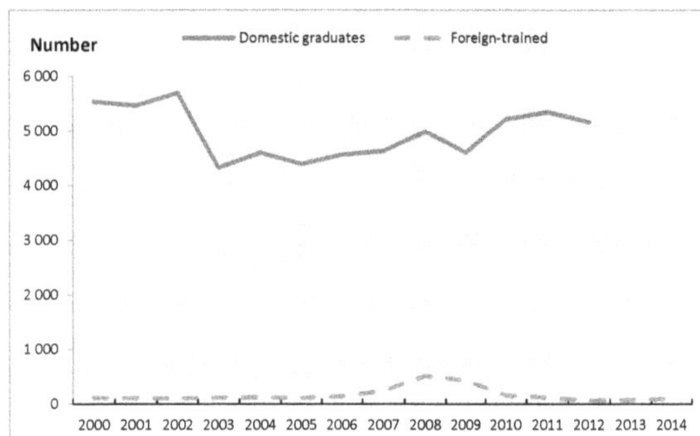

Source: National board of health and Statens Serum Institut.

Doctors, France, 2000-13

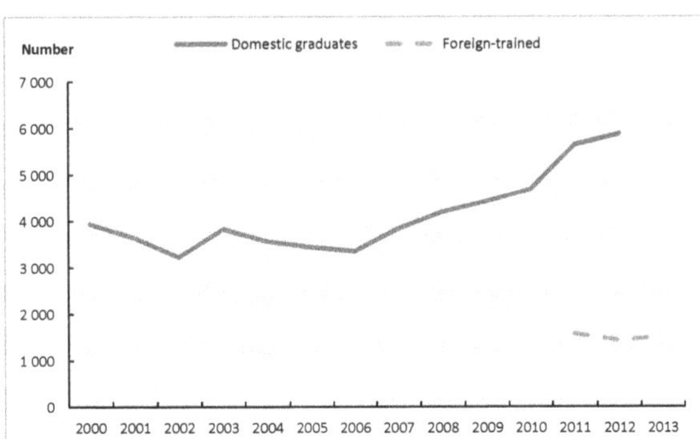

Source: DREES (Ministry of Health) and Ordre des médecins (Medical Council).

Nurses, France, 2000-14

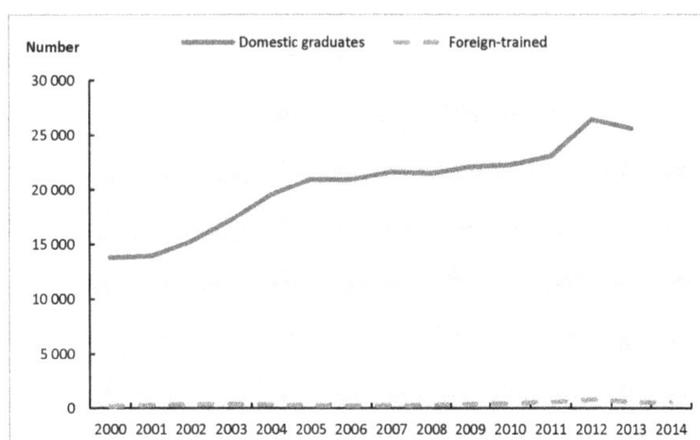

Source: DREES (Ministry of Health).

Figure 4.A2.1. Changes in the number of domestic medical and nursing graduates and inflow of foreign-trained doctors and nurses, selected OECD countries, 2000-14 (or nearest year) *(cont.)*

Doctors, Israel, 2000-14

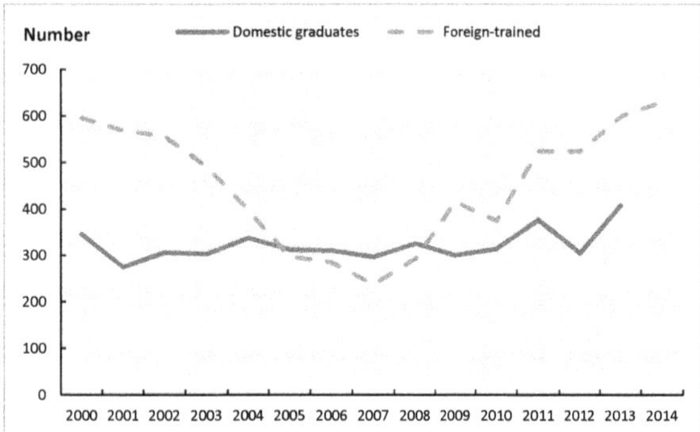

Source: Central Bureau of Statistics and Ministry of Health.

Nurses, Israel, 2000-14

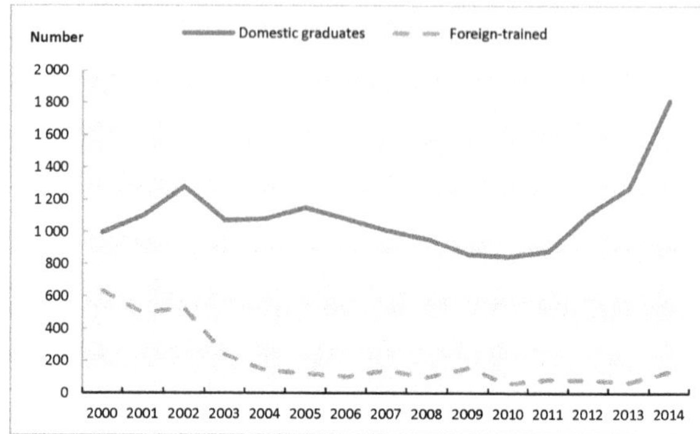

Source: Central Bureau of Statistics and Ministry of Health.

Doctors, Sweden, 2000-13

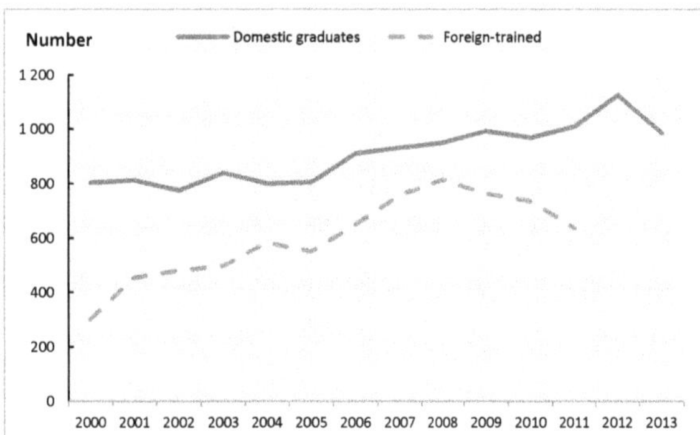

Source: National Board of Health and Welfare.

Nurses, Sweden, 2000-13

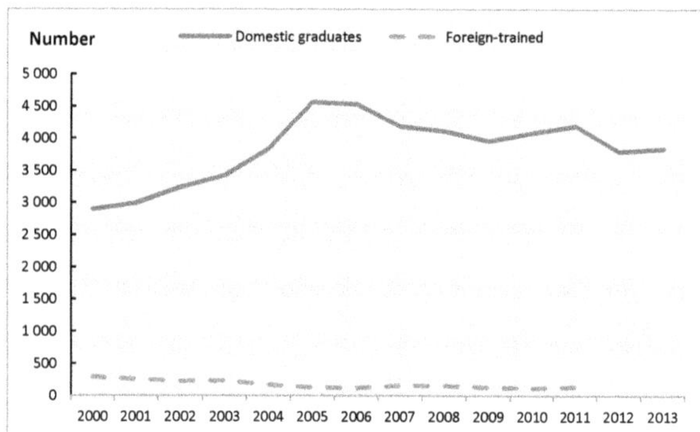

Source: National Board of Health and Welfare.

StatLink http://dx.doi.org/10.1787/888933326396

Chapter 5
Geographic imbalances in the distribution of doctors and health care services in OECD countries

By Tomoko Ono, Michael Schoenstein (formerly from the OECD Health Division) and James Buchan (Queen Margaret University Edinburgh)[1]

The uneven geographic distribution of doctors is one of the most common health workforce policy challenges OECD countries currently face. This chapter provides an overview of this distribution challenge by presenting data on the number of doctors across different regions in OECD countries. It examines the reasons why doctors choose to take up practice in some places, but not in others, and analyses policy responses intended to tackle uneven distribution of doctors. Countries can use three types of strategies, possibly in combination: first, they can aim to select and train future doctors in such a way that they will hopefully distribute more evenly; second, they can try to influence the choice of practice location of new doctors through regulation and financial incentives; and third, they can reform health care delivery in order to be able to provide needed services with fewer doctors by extending the scope of practice of nurses, pharmacists or other providers. Telemedicine is also seen as another increasingly feasible and potentially more efficient option to connect patients and physicians at a distance. While the broad characteristics of these potentially useful interventions can be identified, more robust and regular evaluations are required to determine what policies work to tackle imbalances in physician supply in each context.

5.1. Introduction

Geographic maldistribution of physicians has been a recurring phenomenon and part of health policy discussion for many decades. Nevertheless, the mismatch of physicians to population health in different geographic regions remains one of the most commonly named health workforce policy concerns across OECD countries. According to the *2012-13 OECD Health System Characteristics Survey* most OECD countries consider the maldistribution of doctors to be a key issue to be solved.

The supply of physicians in different localities is most commonly measured in terms of the number of doctors per population (physician density, or physician to population ratio). While the overall physician density has increased substantially in most OECD countries over recent decades, disparities in the density of physicians between different regions still exist in all OECD countries. Typically, rural regions and socio-economically challenged urban regions have lower staffing than more affluent and/or urban ones, and a relatively high level of health worker availability is often observed in capital regions.

Many doctors are reluctant to practise in rural and socio-economically disadvantaged urban regions due to various concerns regarding their career, family and lifestyle. Many countries have tried a variety of incentives or regulations to influence or direct the choice of practice location of physicians. Such policies include medical education, financial incentives, regulation or service delivery reorganisation. While there have been several recent reviews of these policies (Dolea et al., 2010; Bärninghausen and Bloom, 2009), a general lack of follow-up evaluation of their implementation makes it difficult to reach any conclusions about their cost-effectiveness.

The geographic location of physicians will likely continue to be at the forefront of health workforce policy concerns as the population ages. For example, 6% of people over the age of 65 who reported unmet health needs in 2013 indicated that the travel distance and transportation limitations were the main reasons for these unmet care needs in the 28 EU countries. This is expected to be a particular challenge in countries where elderly populations are more concentrated in underserved regions.

This chapter examines factors known to influence physicians' decisions on practice location, and presents a review of policies that have been implemented to address these factors and to improve access to health services in underserved areas. It documents policies with specific attention to characteristics of locality, physicians and the health system.

The chapter begins with a description of the geography of distribution of physician supply (Section 5.2), examining the characteristics of localities of concern. It then turns to investigating factors known to influence physicians' decisions on practice locations (Section 5.3). Section 5.4 proposes a framework for analysis of policy responses. Following this, the chapter details policy responses OECD countries have chosen to tackle maldistribution by focusing on future doctors (Section 5.5), current physicians (Section 5.6) and in doing with less physicians (Section 5.7). Section 5.8 concludes.

5.2. The geography of physician distribution

In many countries, rural regions and socio-economically challenged urban areas are less well-staffed in general and by doctors in particular than other regions, and this may pose a significant barrier for access to health services. OECD countries display very different levels in the total number of practising physicians in the country, ranging from two physicians per 1 000 population or less in Chile and Turkey, to four or more in Austria, Greece and Norway (OECD, 2015). Whatever the overall density of physicians, in all OECD countries, it varies across regions (Figure 5.1).

Figure 5.1. Physician density, by Territorial Level 2 regions, 2013 (or nearest year)

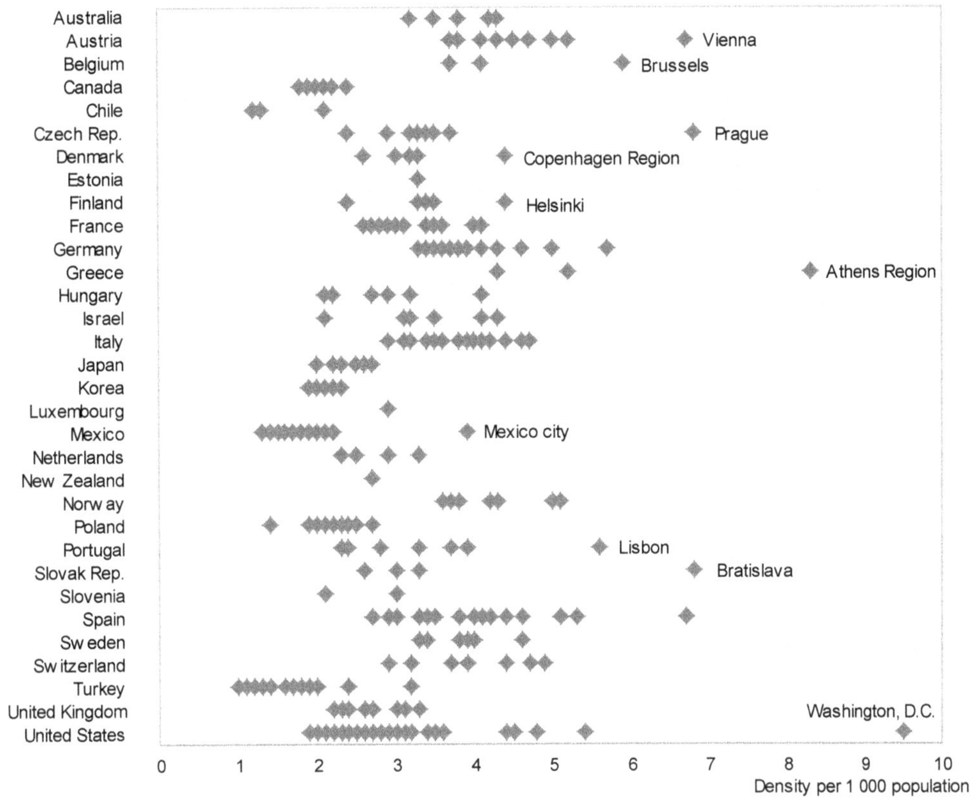

Note: Each observation (point) represents a territorial level 2 region (for example, *region* in France, *Länder* in Germany or *State* in the United States) in each country. The data for Chile relate to 2009 and do not reflect the increase in the number of physicians since then.

Source: OECD (2015), *Health at a Glance 2015: OECD Indicators,* OECD Publishing, Paris, http://dx.doi.org/10.1787/health_glance-2015-en.

StatLink http://dx.doi.org/10.1787/888933326402

Rural regions

Across OECD countries, the number of physicians per capita (i.e. density of physicians) is consistently greater in urban regions, reflecting the concentration of specialist and tertiary services such as surgery, and the preference of specialised practitioners and physicians to practise in urban settings. However, the extent of divergence of density between urban and rural areas varies between countries. Differences in physician density between predominantly urban and rural regions are highest in the Slovak Republic, the Czech Republic and Greece, while the gap is less pronounced in Japan, Korea and Turkey (Figure 5.2).

Figure 5.2. Physicians density in predominantly urban and rural regions, selected countries, 2011 (or nearest year)

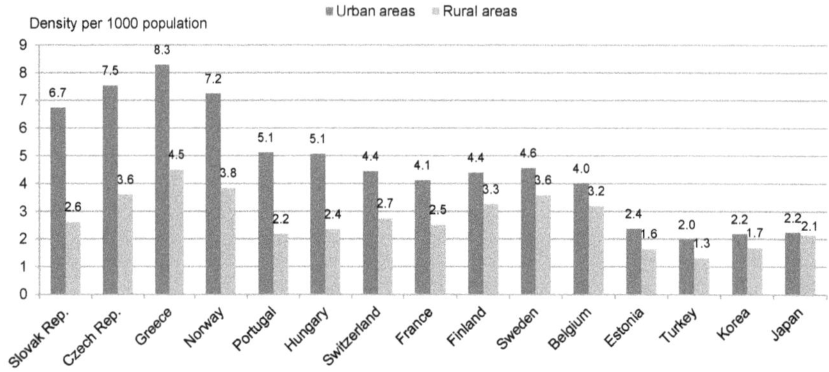

Source: OECD (2015), *Health at a Glance 2015: OECD Indicators,* OECD Publishing, Paris, http://dx.doi.org/10.1787/health_glance-2015-en.

StatLink http://dx.doi.org/10.1787/888933326414

By definition, rural regions have relatively few inhabitants who are widely dispersed. Nevertheless, rural regions significantly differ across OECD countries in population density. The *OECD Regional Database* shows that in Australia and Canada, population density of predominantly rural regions[2] is less than ten inhabitants per km^2 while predominantly rural regions in Germany, Japan and Korea have at least 100 inhabitants per km^2 (Figure 5.3). Hence, whilst lower population density is a universal characteristic of rural areas, it is important to keep in mind that the extent and characteristics of "rurality" can vary markedly across countries, which may limit the transferability of policy options.

Figure 5.3. Population density in predominantly rural areas, inhabitants per km², 2012 (or nearest year)

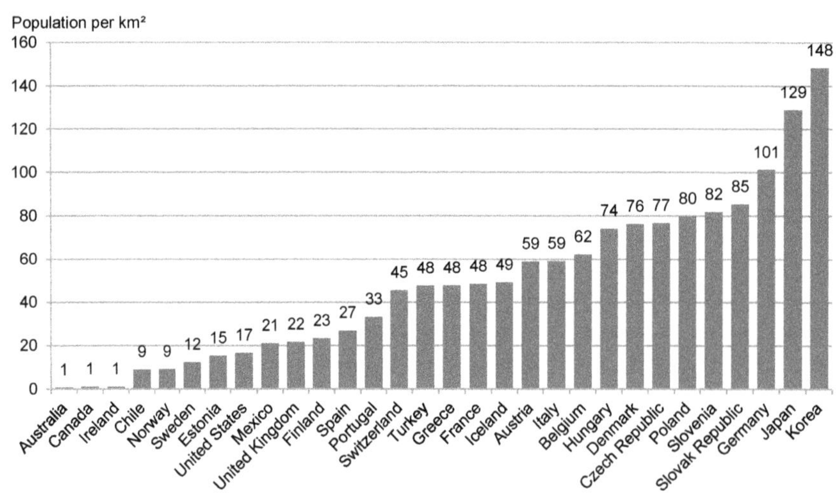

Source: Based on OECD Regional Database (2013), http://dx.doi.org/10.1787/region-data-en.

StatLink http://dx.doi.org/10.1787/888933326423

Low population density makes rural regions a challenging environment for health service provision, as for any other service industries requiring direct "face-to-face" contact with consumers. There are several elements to this impact of rurality.

- First, because populations are dispersed and transport infrastructures often limited, the distance and travel time to the nearest point of service are usually much longer than in urban areas.
- Second, low density rural populations often lack the critical mass and concentration required for efficient location of specialist services.
- Third, because low population density also often means low number of health care providers, this small number of local providers also implies that staffing mix options may be limited, and there may also be staffing constraints over 24/7 service provision.
- Fourth, there is a requirement in many small rural and remote communities for general practitioners to have an additional skill set, such as obstetrics, emergency care and surgery.

Some countries also make a distinction between "rural" and "remote" in terms of service provision and workforce availability. For example, in Australia, "it needs to be emphasised that whilst the rural and remote sectors have some issues in common, there are also some stark differences. The biggest, for example, is the relative absence of medical practitioners in remote areas. Remote health is predominantly reliant on the core workforce of Aboriginal and Torres Strait Islander health workers, and practitioners and remote area nurses (RANs) with support from a range of multi-disciplinary health professionals across the fly-in/fly-out (FIFO) and drive-in/drive-out (DIDO) allied health and medical professions" (Health Workforce Australia, 2013). In Scotland, "rural and remote" covers low density populations in the mainland highlands, where transport infrastructure is limited, but also includes population clusters on many small islands only accessible by boat or plane. In Japan, the designation of "isolated rural areas (*hekichi*)" also takes into account natural terrain and climate (islands and mountainous areas with heavy snow) that create a hindrance to accessing necessary services.

Disadvantaged urban and suburban regions

While the distance to a physician's location of work is a dominant factor determining access to health services in rural areas, the factors creating barriers to access in urban disadvantaged areas can be less obvious, and perhaps more complex. People who live in disadvantaged urban and suburban regions may have distinctly different educational, economic, cultural, and demographic backgrounds from their more affluent neighbours. Inhabitants of disadvantaged urban areas tend to have a worse health status and thus potentially higher demand for health services. Moreover, their life circumstances require health care providers who understand their health needs and social conditions and can provide appropriate care.

As the first point of access to health care, it is ideal for a GP-based service or family health practice to be in their community and understand their needs and health condition. However, socio-economically disadvantaged urban areas often have difficulties attracting physicians. For example, in Paris, the density of GPs ranged in 2009 from 3.2 per 1 000 population in the (wealthy) 8th *arrondissement* (city district) to 0.8 GPs per 1 000 population in the (poor) 20th *arrondissement*. Differences in densities are even more pronounced if compared to the surrounding *départements* (districts). In socio-economically disadvantaged areas in Seine-Saint-Denis, the general density is much lower, with only 0.4 GPs per 1 000 population (URPS Médecins IDF, 2013). In the United States as well, there are shortages of GPs in socio-economically disadvantaged urban areas (Heisler, 2013). In German cities, the share of long-term unemployed people correlates with a lower density of doctors (Greß and Stegemüller, 2011).

5.3. Influences on location choice of doctors

Many different factors play a role in a physician's decision to practise in a certain region: 1) the general *attractiveness of the location environment*, including educational options for children, career opportunities for spouses as well as personal safety concerns, housing and access to cultural activities; 2) the *mode of employment*, determining the options physicians have when they enter the labour market or wish to take up a new position; 3) the *income potential*, which is likely to be influenced by payment schemes and volume of activities; 4) their *working conditions*, including working hours, access to appropriate medical equipment and support services, and career and professional development opportunities; 5) *prestige and recognition*, as many medical students and physicians appear to value less general medicine and rural medicine; and 6) medical students' *background and expectations* of work and life in underserved regions and their capacity to adjust to rural or socio-economically challenged regions.

General environment

Socio-economically disadvantaged urban areas and rural regions are often considered to be less attractive environments to live in. In rural areas, less developed infrastructure, limited children's educational opportunities or limited spouses' career opportunities can reduce attractiveness.

In qualitative surveys of family medicine graduates in Canada, lifestyle issues and family obligations were listed as some of the main reasons for not practising in rural areas, along with other work concerns (Lu et al., 2008). Similarly, a study in Germany cites that few leisure facilities are a negative aspect of rural practice (Natanzon et al., 2010). However, this is also a matter of physicians' personal preferences, and the type of "leisure facility" that matters may vary significantly. For some physicians, the rurality of a location may be an attraction in itself. For example, a survey from Colorado (United States) reports that 70% of rural physicians respond that recreational or leisure activity was one of the very important factors in keeping them in rural settings (Colorado Health Institute, 2012).

Mode of employment

The mode of employment of doctors may also influence greatly their choice of practice location. For example, where doctors are salaried employees, such as in Finland, their choice of practice location is determined to a large extent by the availability of job vacancies in any given region. Financial incentives can also be added to influence practice location. Where physicians are predominantly publicly employed, the government may have the scope to directly pay bonuses or vary salaries according to location. Where physicians are predominantly self-employed and capitation agreements or fee-for-service schedules are the basis of remuneration, these mechanisms can be regionally diversified or weighted, or additional incentives may need to be offered in order to provide sufficient financial incentives to recruit and retain staff in rural/underserved areas (see Section 5.6).

The *2012-13 OECD Health System Characteristics Survey* provides an overview of the predominant mode of employment of doctors in various OECD countries. In 19 countries that reported this information, general practitioners (GPs) are self-employed or privately employed. However, in Finland, Israel, Portugal, Slovenia, Spain and Sweden, general practitioners are publicly employed. For specialists working in ambulatory care, the picture is similar, although there are more countries where they are publicly employed (Tables 5.1 and 5.2).

Table 5.1. General practitioners: Predominant mode of employment, OECD countries

Self-employed	Privately employed	Publicly employed
Austria	Australia	Finland
Belgium	Poland	Israel
Canada	United States	Portugal
Czech Republic		Slovenia
Denmark		Spain
France		Sweden
Germany		
Greece		
Ireland		
Italy		
Korea		
Netherlands		
New Zealand		
Norway		
Switzerland		
United Kingdom		

Source: 2012-13 OECD Health System Characteristics Survey, http://www.oecd.org/els/health-systems/characteristics.htm.

Table 5.2. Specialists in ambulatory care: Predominant mode of employment, OECD countries

Self-employed	Privately employed	Publicly employed
Austria	Australia	Denmark
Belgium		Finland
Canada		Ireland
Czech Republic		Israel
France		Italy
Germany		New Zealand
Greece		Norway
Iceland		Portugal
Korea		Slovenia
Netherlands		Spain
Poland		Sweden
Switzerland		United Kingdom
United States		

Source: 2012-13 OECD Health System Characteristics Survey, http://www.oecd.org/els/health-systems/characteristics.htm.

Opportunities for “dual practice”, where doctors hold two jobs, in many cases in the public and private sector, may also influence their geographic distribution. Significant private sector earning opportunities are more likely to be available in higher-density urban areas than in rural areas, thereby possibly influencing the choice of practice location. As such, perceptions of limited dual practice opportunities may be another factor in deterring doctors to locate to areas of low population density or with relatively poor populations. The impact of dual practice varies among countries, based on its extent and the presence or absence of regulatory policies (Table 5.3). There are three main categories of dual practice regulation mechanisms that have been used across OECD countries: 1) total banning of dual practice; 2) allowing dual practice with restrictions; and 3) allowing dual practice without restrictions.

Table 5.3. Reported dual practice regulation in OECD countries

Always allowed	Allowed in certain cases	Not allowed
Austria	Canada	Germany
Belgium	Greece	Hungary
Chile	Iceland	Ireland
Czech Republic	Italy	Korea
Denmark	Japan	Luxembourg
Finland	Poland	Sweden
France	Portugal	
Israel	Slovenia	
Mexico	Spain	
Netherlands	United States	
New Zealand		
Norway		
Switzerland		
United Kingdom		

Source: 2012-13 OECD Health System Characteristics Survey, http://www.oecd.org/els/health-systems/characteristics.htm.

Income potential

In fee-for-service systems or capitation systems, the number of services a doctor provides or the number of patients a physician has on his/her patient list directly impacts income. Without financial adjustments in the payment scheme, physicians in rural and disadvantaged areas may in theory earn less than colleagues who practise elsewhere because they might provide a lower volume of services or have a lower number of patients.

However, in practice, available data from five countries show that the unadjusted (for workload or working hours) income of GPs or primary care physicians was at least similar or higher in rural areas compared to those working in urban areas. In Australia, France and Germany, work-related incomes of rural physicians were about 10% to 15% higher than those in urban regions, and in the United States the difference was about 6% higher. In Norway, the incomes were roughly equal (Figure 5.4).

Still, any slight advantage in terms of income may not be sufficient to compensate for other perceived disadvantages of GPs and other primary care physicians to work in rural areas. This may therefore not be sufficient to address the issue of maldistribution.

Figure 5.4. Average annual income of GPs or primary care physicians, rural/urban ratios, selected OECD countries

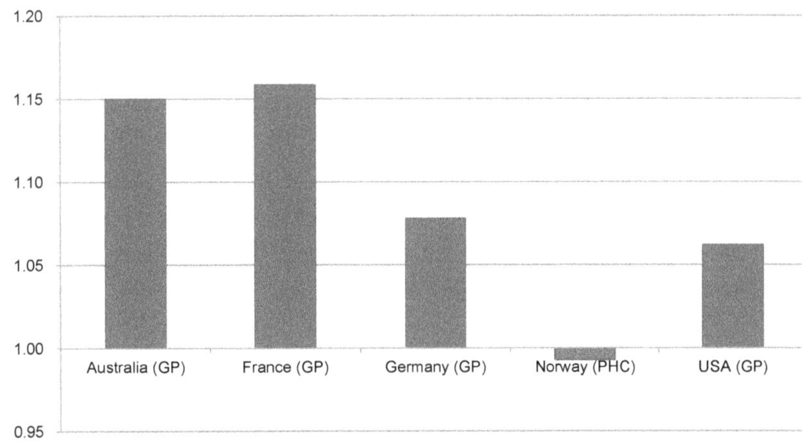

Source: Australia: Cheng et al. (2010), income, major cities vs. outer regional, rural and remote; France: DREES (2013), income, predominantly urban area vs. predominantly rural using OECD definition, data provided to the OECD; Germany: von Stillfried (2012), revenue major cities vs. rural areas. Norway: Deloitte (2011), income, cities with more than 50 000 inhabitants vs. the rest of the country; United States: Weeks and Wallace (2008), income, metropolitan areas vs. non-metropolitan areas.

StatLink http://dx.doi.org/10.1787/888933326432

Working conditions

Rural GPs in some countries work significantly more hours than their urban colleagues (Figure 5.5).

Figure 5.5. Average weekly hours worked by GPs/Family physicians, urban vs. rural regions, selected OECD countries

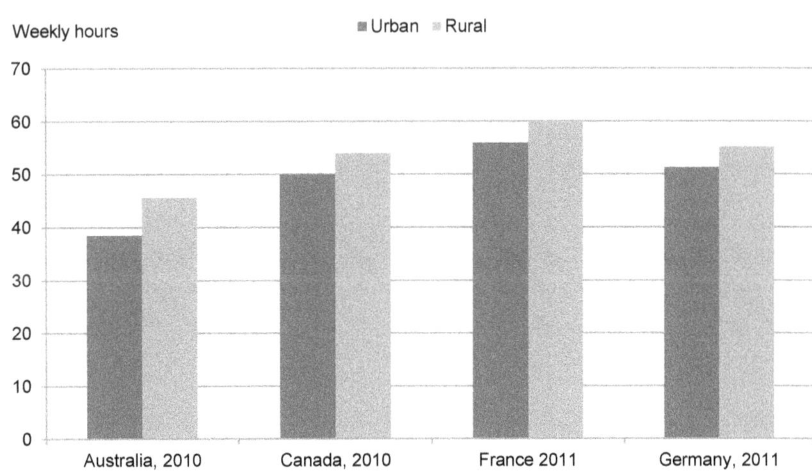

Source: Australia: McGrail et al. (2012), major cities vs. outer regional, rural, and remote; Canada: Buske (2012), urban area vs. rural area which include small town, rural and geographically isolated/remote area; France: Jakoubovitch et al. (2012), urban vs. rural areas based on INSEE definition; Germany: Steinhäuser et al. (2011), urban vs. rural area based on the level of rurality rated by physicians.

StatLink http://dx.doi.org/10.1787/888933326449

The traditional view of "one physician, alone, always at work, always on call" (Elliott, 2012) summarises doctors' concerns about rural conditions. Doctors in solo practices may have no other physician in near proximity, facing significant time on call (Elliott, 2012; Natanzon et al., 2010). The inability to have uninterrupted time away from work may cause significant stress (Sim, 2011). In Australia, McGrail et al. (2012) found that combined working and on-call time for doctors in medium-sized, small and very small rural communities was on average a third to double of that of metropolitan doctors in 2010.

Other aspects of working conditions also play a role in decisions to practice in disadvantaged urban areas. In France, physicians working in such areas report language problems, difficulties in interacting with patients from different cultural backgrounds and security concerns as some of the day-to-day issues they are facing (ONM, 2012).

Prestige and recognition

The relative prestige and status of medical jobs, specialties and work locations can also influence physicians' choice of practice location. Rural practice has relatively low prestige in some countries. In Australia, Creed, Searle and Rogers (2010) found that while many specialties rank high in lifestyle or prestige (e.g., high prestige but bad lifestyle for surgery; low prestige and good lifestyle for public health medicine), rural medicine is ranked low for prestige and lifestyle among medical students (Figure 5.6). Other studies have indicated that Australian medical students and physicians who place less value on prestige and status are more likely to have worked in rural areas or intend to do so (Conomos et al., 2013).

Figure 5.6. Ranking of prestige and lifestyle of physician specialty, Australian medical students

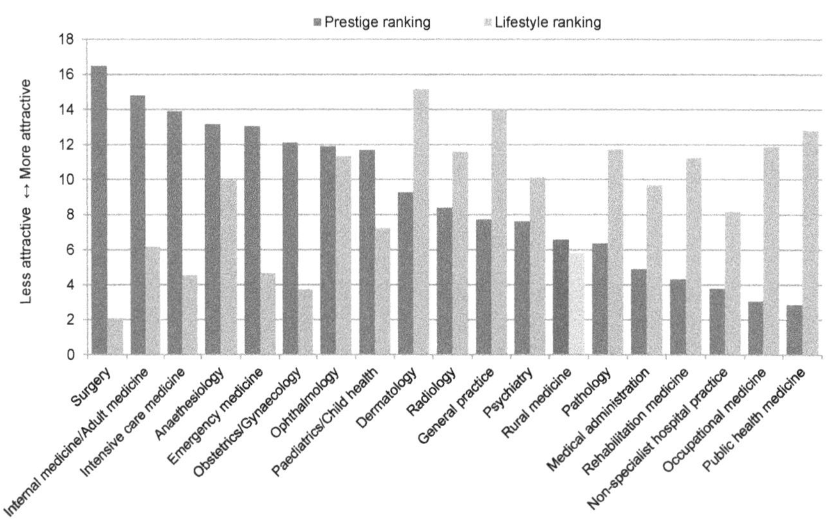

Source: Based on data presented in Creed, P.A., J. Searle and M.E. Rogers (2010), "Medical Specialty Prestige and Lifestyle Preferences for Medical Students", *Social Science and Medicine*, Vol. 71, No. 6, pp. 1084-1088, September.

StatLink http://dx.doi.org/10.1787/888933326454

But physicians' career choice may also be influenced by the recognition of their work contribution from peers and the community they serve. In a US survey of osteopathic students and residents, 70% of medical students and 78% of residents considered rural practice to have greater community impact (Colegrove and Whitacre, 2009).

Origin and experience

The background of doctors and to what extent their expectations of practice in an underserved region match the reality may also influence their location choice. If work experiences in specific locations during their training period were positive or negative, this may alter of course their decisions. A German study found that medical students' expectations of work in rural settings are much worse than the reality. Unsurprisingly, this coincides with a clear preference for practice in urban areas among medical graduates (Gibis et al., 2012).

Several studies have considered the link between a physician's origin and the likelihood of choosing rural practice (Laven and Wilkinson, 2003; Wilson et al., 2009). A physician's rural origin is often reported as a determinant of future choice to practice in rural areas (Hancock et al., 2009). In the United States, Rabinowitz et al. (2011) examined why the Physicians Shortage Area Program (PSAP) of Jefferson Medical College in Pennsylvania (a programme targeted to produce rural family practice physicians) has been effective and demonstrated that rural upbringing and interest for family practice in the first year explain its success. Similarly, a study in Australia demonstrated that the number of years spent in a rural area prior to entering a medical school is a good predictor for practising in a rural area for GPs and specialists (McGrail et al., 2011; Figure 5.7). The strength of a rural background as a factor in determining rural practice for physicians was also supported in studies in Canada, Japan and South Africa (Laven and Wilkinson, 2003; Wilson et al., 2009; Matsumoto et al., 2008; Feldman et al., 2008). Consequently, training physicians with a rural background has been advocated as a solution to filling vacancies in underserved rural regions (see Section 5.5).

Figure 5.7. Differential effect of physician background on the probability of working in rural areas, Australia and the United States

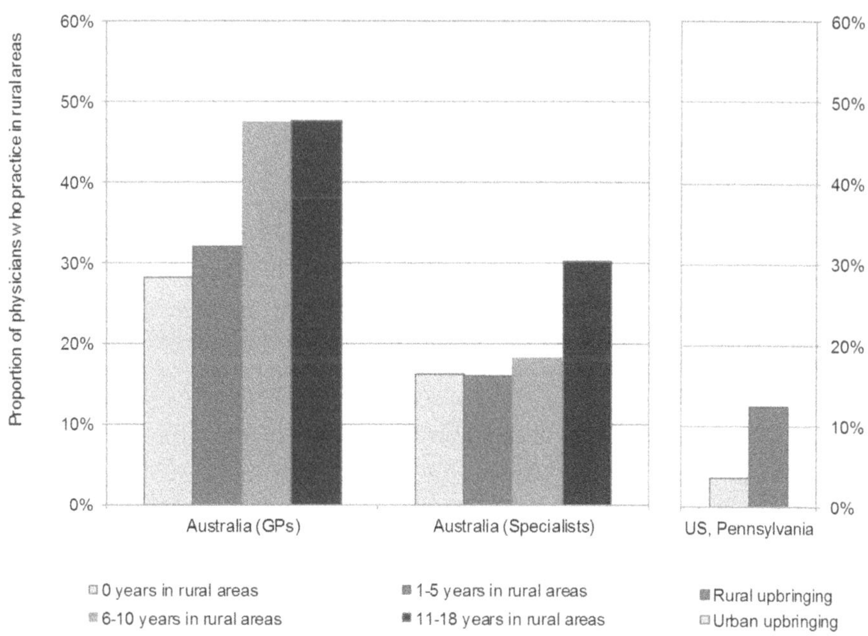

Source: Australia: McGrail et al. (2011); United States: Rabinowitz et al. (2011).

StatLink http://dx.doi.org/10.1787/888933326469

5.4. Policy strategies and areas for action

Following Bennett and Philips (2010), at any point during their training and career, physicians can be grouped into: 1) those committed to practise in underserved regions; 2) those who may be interested, with the right incentives; and 3) those who are not interested. Physicians' preferences may change throughout their career. Policy makers may have multiple points of intervention across a doctor's professional lifespan to influence their decision. In addition, health service delivery may also be re-designed to serve local communities with fewer physicians on site.

Based on the classifications proposed in a number of international literature reviews (Jones et al., 2012; Dolea et al., 2010; Wilson et al., 2009; Bourgueil et al., 2006), policies can be grouped in four distinct areas of action, which are not mutually exclusive and can complement each other:

- First, through interventions at different points in the **medical education** process, policies may influence the choice of practice location at the end of the training period. These include the selection of students in *entry to medical schools* and the design and geographic distribution of *post-graduate clinical training* programmes.
- Second, countries can offer various types of **financial incentives** to attract more physicians in underserved areas, starting from providing special scholarship at *entry to medical schools* and/or *post-graduate clinical training* (possibly combined with return-of-service obligation), to *one-off payments* to doctors to support their installation in underserved areas, to recurrent payments and bonuses to recruit and retain them in underserved areas.
- Third, countries may **regulate** which type of physicians is allowed to work where. Regulation can be put in place at the time of *entry to post-graduate clinical training* (e.g. in the form of return-of-service agreements) or in restricting the choice of practice location when *new doctors want to set up a first practice*.
- Fourth, a **re-design in health service delivery** may help to improve the working conditions of doctors in underserved areas (e.g., by creating group practices to overcome the isolation of solo practice) and/or promote the use of innovative health service delivery to provide adequate level of access with fewer physicians (e.g. through telemedicine or shifting some health service provision from physicians to other local health care providers).

5.5. Targeting future doctors: Medical education policies

A number of policies can help attract more medical students who will end up working in underserved regions. These policies generally aim to encourage more people from rural and underserved communities to pursue medical careers and/or reduce or remove barriers created by negative expectations of practice in rural or disadvantaged urban areas.

The extent to which countries control access to medical education influences the policy space governments have to design incentives for medical students to work in underserved areas. Nearly all OECD countries restrict in one way or the other entry into initial medical education and/or entry into post-graduate specialty training (see Chapter 3 for more information).

The way in which the costs of medical education are shared between public and private payers is another factor influencing the potential use and effectiveness of this policy lever. Where students bear a higher share of the costs, targeted scholarship or debt subsidy programmes may be more effective in influencing their practice location than in countries where there are no tuition fees.

Policies aimed at student selection

In Australia, the federal government offers three medical school placement schemes, although the third one (the MRBS) has been closed to new entrants in 2016. Under the commonwealth-supported places scheme, students pay part of the medical degree and the remainder is subsidised by the government, with no conditions attached. Both the Bonded Medical Places (BMP) scheme and the Medical Rural Bonded Scholarship (MRBS) scheme require students to repay the cost to the government of their place (BMP) or their scholarship (MRBS) if they break the contract. In the case of the MRBS scheme, physicians may not be able to have access to the Medicare schedule for up to 12 years.

Under the BMP scheme, the Australian Government offers an additional 700 medical training placements per year (rising to 800 from 2017). Students have to sign a deed of agreement with the government to work in a district of physician shortage for a period equal to the length of training. A 2013 review (Mason, 2013) noted that more than 4 500 participants had such an agreement at that time, but only one had commenced his/her return-of-service obligation and three had chosen to repay the cost of their education. In contrast, students offered the MRBS scheme received substantial financial aid and signed a contract with the government to work in a rural or remote area for six years after completing specialist training. There were 100 placements available each year. Since 2001, more than 1 200 students participated in this programme but only 50 have started the return-of-service obligation period. The MRBS scheme was closed to new from 2016, with these 100 medical places being transferred to the MRBS scheme (Department of Health, 2015).

Japanese medical schools have a regional quota system of student selection to increase the number of doctors within each prefecture. Under the "one prefecture, one medical school" policy of 1973, the 47 prefectures have each had at least one medical school since 1981. While the numbers of medical schools and training spots are centrally controlled and have barely changed in the last three decades, each university can create its own student selection criteria and give recruitment incentives. The regional quota systems mainly involve offering a scholarship with a term-defined practice requirement (6-9 years), through: selection for medical school entry from within the same prefectures in which the school is located, or selection of students willing to serve in regional services, regardless of their origin, or the offer of a conditional scholarship for those already in medical school. In 1997, only two medical schools had a regional quota system covering 11 students. By 2014, 68 of 79 schools offered regional quota spots, for 1 452 students (16% of the total intake, see Figure 5.8).

Figure 5.8. Regional quota in Japan, 1997-2014

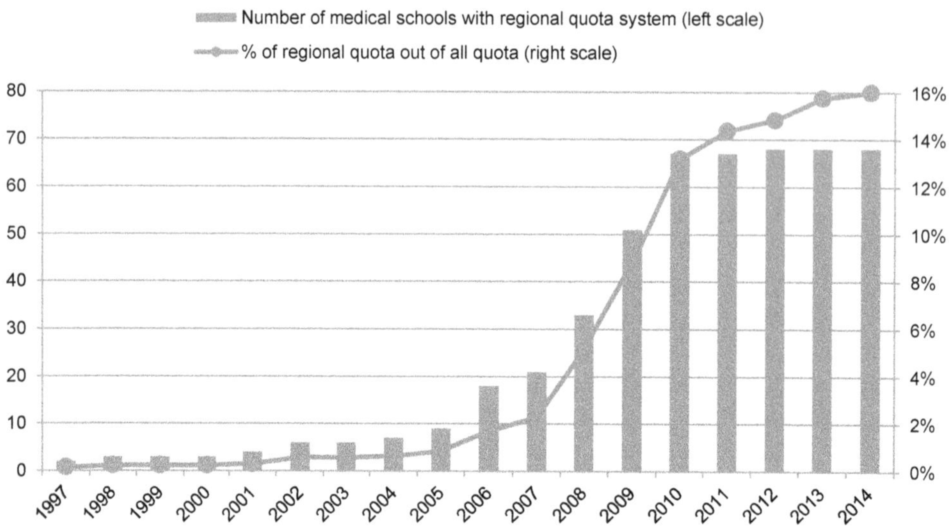

Source: Medical Education Division, Ministry of Education, Culture, Sports, Science and Technology (MEXT), 2015.

StatLink http://dx.doi.org/10.1787/888933326473

A 2011 Ministry of Education, Culture, Sports, Science and Technology (MEXT) study covering six medical schools with regional-quota medical graduates showed that 89% of regional-quota graduates have remained within their prefecture, compared with 54% only of normal-entry graduates.

Policies aimed at training institutions

Some countries have used two often complementary options to re-design the supply of medical education and training places to achieve a better geographic distribution of doctors: 1) setting up medical schools to train students specifically in underserved (rural) regions; and 2) increasing the number of specialty training places outside universities and hospitals and into ambulatory settings in underserved areas.

In Norway, the University of Tromsø's school of medicine was established in 1972 in northern Norway to address a chronic shortage of physicians. When the school was established, a quota of 25% was reserved for students from northern Norway in the belief that a greater percentage of these students would remain there after graduation; this share was increased to 50% in 1979 and 60% in 1998 (Alexandersen et al., 2004). As a result, the number of medical graduates with a north-Norwegian origin increased from 41% in the period from 1979 to 1988, to 57% in the period from 1996 to 2001. Research has shown that most medical graduates from the University of Tromsø do remain in northern Norway. Of the medical students who graduated between 1979 and 1988, 56% continued to work in northern Norway, though this fell to 51% for graduates from 1996 to 2001. There is also evidence that the likelihood of graduates remaining in northern Norway is particularly high if they are of northern Norwegian origin. Among the University of Tromsø graduates from 1996 to 2001, 75% of physicians with northern Norwegian origin chose to practise there, while only 19% of physicians with a southern Norwegian origin remained after graduation (Alexandersen et al., 2004).

Japan's Jichi Medical University was also established in 1972 with the sole purpose of training physicians for areas with insufficient doctors. The university is technically private, but is managed by an educational foundation, and co-funded by 47 prefectural governments and the national government. Each prefecture chooses local high school graduates for admission, and the university undertakes a second screening, with eventually two or three students entering the university each year. After six years of medical training, students are obliged to return to their prefecture of origin for practice. Students are exempt from repaying the loans they receive in medical school if they work in public hospitals, designated by the prefectural governor, for a period equivalent to two-thirds of the period during which they receive a student loan (this is called the "obligatory period"). By 2015, 96% of graduate physicians (a total of 3 910) had completed or were completing their obligatory period. The retention rate of graduates in their home prefectures beyond the time of their service obligation was around 70%. Graduates that fulfil their service requirement are more likely to practise in a rural area than graduates from other medical schools. Inoue, Matsumoto and Sawada (2007) have shown that even after completion of their service obligation, the share of Jichi graduates practising in rural areas is significantly higher.

In Canada, the Northern Ontario School of Medicine (NOSM), a joint initiative of two rural universities more than 1 000 km apart, welcomed its first medical students in 2005. This School actively seeks to recruit local students or those from similar northern, rural, remote, Aboriginal, or francophone backgrounds. Clinical education takes place in local communities and health service settings, with 70 teaching and research sites. Students who choose a rural area to practise after their training are eligible for funding from a loan-repayment programme. While it is too early to assess the long-term impacts of this initiative, about 70% of graduates are training in family medicine, mostly in rural regions.

5.6. Targeting current doctors: Carrots and sticks

Another strategy is to target current doctors to increase the number of physicians in underserved regions. This may include "carrots and sticks" – financial incentives and suitable regulatory measures.

Financial incentives

Many countries have introduced financial incentives, as shown in Table 5.4, to encourage more physicians to practice in rural or socio-economically disadvantaged urban areas.

Financial incentives can compensate for longer working hours or a less advantageous "business environment" for doctors in underserved areas. The evaluation of the effect of financial incentives is difficult, as they are often part of a package with various incentives, and physicians may receive multiple financial incentives from different sources at the same time. It is difficult (and unadvisable) to design financial incentives that target only those willing to move to underserved areas because of financial incentives. It may incur "wastage" by providing incentives to those who would have practised in underserved areas regardless of government intervention (Bärninghausen and Bloom, 2009; Dolea et al., 2010).

Table 5.4. Reported financial incentives to foster a better geographic distribution of physicians

Incentives in place	No incentives reported
Australia	Austria
Belgium	Czech Republic
Canada	Iceland
Chile	Ireland
Denmark (Regions)	Italy
Finland	Japan
France	Luxembourg
Germany	Netherlands
Greece	Poland
Hungary	Spain
Israel	
Korea	
Mexico	
New Zealand	
Norway	
Portugal	
Slovenia	
Sweden	
Switzerland	
United States	
United Kingdom (England and Wales)	

Source: 2012-13 OECD Health System Characteristics Survey; National Audit Office, United Kingdom (2008).

Non-wage-related payments (one-off payment)

Non-wage-related payments are used to encourage physicians to move to or stay in underserved areas. These are often "up-front payments" intended to help facilitate a location choice, or are conditional on the criteria being met, which may be based on practice size or volume of activity.

Several countries have implemented non-wage-related incentives targeting various stages of physicians' careers. Many policies target physicians opening their practice for the first time. In Germany, 11 out of 16 states (*Länder*) offer financial incentives for GPs opening their practice for the first time. GPs can receive a payment for opening a practice in underserved areas. Subsidies range from EUR 15 000 to EUR 60 000 depending on the state, degree of shortage, municipality size, and types of services provided. Costs are either shared between the state government, the association of statutory health insurance physicians and insurance companies, or borne entirely by one of these stakeholders. In some states, the one-time payment comes with a return-of-service obligation of five to ten years. There is no evaluation as to whether it has helped recruitment.

Similar policies exist in Canadian provinces. In Ontario, the Northern and Rural Recruitment and Retention Initiative offers grants of between CAD 80 000 and CAD 117 600 for a practice opening in a rural area (HPM, 2008).

Wage-related financial incentives (recurrent payment)

Physicians in underserved areas sometimes receive financial incentives linked to income. Some target particular life stages where critical decisions for practice location are made. These payments aim to compensate rural GPs for a smaller number of patients and/or longer working hours.

Across OECD countries, a variety of payment mechanisms exist across a range of institutional arrangements (Table 5.5). Physicians work in different settings, such as solo or group practices or health centres, where they may be salaried or self-employed. Payments may be directed to institutions, in the case of health centres or group practices, or directly to physicians providing services, or both.

Financial incentives can be arranged along with the existing payment structure to target specific physicians and their performance. Payments to institutions comprise global budgets that define a maximum expenditure in a given time period (and often region), capitation agreements that pay providers in function of the number of patients enrolled in their practice, independent of service provision, fee-for-service arrangements that pay for each service provided, or pay-for–performance (P4P) arrangements that make at least part of a payment conditional on reaching certain objectives. Payments to individual physicians comprise salaries, capitation agreements, fee-for-service schedules and other arrangements including P4P schemes.

In countries where physicians work predominantly in solo and group practices, there is almost always an element of fee-for-service payments and some capitation-based payments. In countries where physicians work in health centres, salaries play a much more important role.

Table 5.5. Summary of payment mechanisms for primary care physicians and institutions

Type of predominant institution of primary care	Countries	Payment of institutions					Payment of physicians			
		Global budget	Capitation	Fee-for-service	Pay-for-performance	Other	Salaried	Capitation	Fee-for-service	Other (incl. P4P)
Doctors in solo practice	Germany*								X	
	Austria*								X	
	Belgium*							X	X	
	Korea*	Non applicable							X	X
	France*								X	X
	Greece*								X	
	Czech Rep.							X	X	X
	Switzerland*							X	X	
Public centres	Spain		X		X		X	X		X
	Finland	X					X		X	
	Iceland	X					X			
	Portugal	X	X		X		X			
	Sweden		X	X	X		X			
Group practice with doctors and other health professionals	Australia			X	X				X	X
	Denmark		X	X				X	X	
	Ireland		X					X		
	Netherlands*	X	X	X	X			X	X	X
	New Zealand		X	X	X		X	X	X	
	Norway		X	X				X	X	
	United Kingdom		X	X	X	X		X	X	X
	Poland*		X					X		
Group practices with only doctors	Canada		X	X		X	X	X	X	
	Italy		X						X	X

* Social insurance systems.

Source: 2012-13 OECD Health System Characteristics Survey.

Basic income guarantees may work as an incentive for physicians at the point in time when they set up a practice in an underserved region. In France, some recently qualified GPs benefit from a guaranteed annual income of EUR 82 800. This measure was introduced in 2013 and is available annually to 500 GPs and time-limited to the first two years of practice (Ministère des Affaires sociales et de la Santé, 2015). In Denmark, similar revenue guarantees are in place in Northern Jutland and the Capital Region based on a fixed list size. If GPs have not enlisted 1 600 patients, the government provides DKK 1 500 per "missing" patient for two years until 1 600 patients are reached. In the Capital region, this policy is linked with a five-year return-of-service obligation. GPs are also compensated for taking over patients who have lost their GP due to closures. In Northern Jutland, GPs receive a higher remuneration if they sign up more than 1 760 patients. The revenue for additional patients is doubled (PLO, 2013).

Other financial incentives can compensate for challenging work conditions. In the Canadian province of British Columbia, the Rural Retention Programme grants physicians an annual bonus based on "isolation points" determined by the existence of other physicians in surrounding areas and the community's geographic characteristics. In 2008, 144 communities were entitled to grant physicians an allowance and 1 568 physicians benefitted in 2007-08 (Ministry of Health of British Columbia, 2012).

Financial incentives can aim to encourage doctors to postpone retirement. In Canada's rural areas in Alberta, annual bonuses range from CAD 4 000 after five years of practice, rising to CAD 10 000 after 26 years (HPM, 2008). In Denmark's Northern Jutland, GPs receive DKK 55 000 per quarter between the ages of 62 and 65 (PLO, 2013). In the German state of Thuringia, GPs aged 65 and above can receive EUR 1 500 per quarter, in addition to their normal revenues, for working in underserved rural areas (AOK, 2011).

In summary, financial incentives may compensate for some of the disadvantages of service in less attractive regions, rendering it more economically attractive. While they may be necessary to level the playing field, they are no "game changer" for location choice. While doctors in underserved regions can receive higher payments, staff levels in these regions generally have remained lower. Financial incentives may be more effective in channelling money to physicians in underserved regions but less effective at attracting new recruits. Investment in financial incentives should be considered carefully on merit.

Regulatory policies

Regulatory measures can foster a better distribution of physicians and restrict or direct the choice of practice location. There are two main ways countries may set up such regulations:

- *Regulations of practice location*: there may be *de-facto* limitations using system features to limit location choice, or inducing a better distribution through legislation, for example by allowing new practices to open only where the physician density is below a certain threshold.
- *Targeting international medical graduates*: countries can make the immigration of foreign-trained doctors, and/or their entry into specialty training, conditional on practice in designated areas.

About 70 countries have experience with some form of regulatory approach, mostly low and middle-income countries (Frehywot et al., 2010). Most OECD countries, however, do not constrain location choice for physicians who want to set up an ambulatory care practice.

In the *2012-13 OECD Health System Characteristics Survey*, four countries reported some de-facto limitations in practice location choice. In Austria, contracts physicians make with social insurance for reimbursement are regionally limited. In the Czech Republic, doctors need to engage in a reimbursement agreement whose availability may be easier in some regions than others. In Finland, health care delivery is organised at the municipal level, so the availability of job vacancies determines a physician's location choice. In the United Kingdom, commissioning arrangements may influence the availability of posts. Denmark, Germany, Norway and Slovenia restrict the choice of location, as do two Canadian provinces (Table 5.6).

One advantage of regulatory approaches is that the direct financial cost is generally limited to administrative costs. Only a few regulatory approaches have been evaluated. Evidence is particularly lacking on the regulatory framework on the basis of some benchmarks, such as a density threshold, to improve physician geographic distribution. Available evidence on the impact of return-of-service agreements, which in some countries target foreign-trained physicians, indicates some placements are effective in the short term, but such policies do not necessarily provide long-term staffing stability to underserved regions (Dywili et al., 2012; Wilson et al., 2009; Han and Humphreys, 2006).

Table 5.6. Reported limitations to the choice of practice location

No restriction of choice of practice location	De facto limitation of choice of practice location	Restricted choice of practice location
Belgium	Austria	Canada (New Brunswick, Quebec)
Canada (except two provinces)	Czech Republic	Denmark
France	Finland	Germany
Greece	United Kingdom	Norway
Ireland		Slovenia
Israel		
Japan		
Korea		
Netherlands		
New Zealand		
Poland		
Portugal		
Spain		
Sweden		
Switzerland		
United States		

Source: 2012-13 OECD Health System Characteristics Survey.

Regulation of practice location

In Germany, the number of practice permits for ambulatory care physicians in a specific region is limited, based on a national service delivery quota. Physicians need to obtain a practice permit to be reimbursed by the statutory health insurance. The number of these permits is controlled by the National Association of Statutory Health Insurance Physicians (NASHIP) through its 17 state associations. The NASHIP is the self-regulated organisation of about 120 000 physicians practising under the statutory health insurance.

It is mandated by the government to guarantee medical service coverage of the population based on a quota agreed within the self-administration of the German health care system. The service coverage is measured based on the ratio between physicians and inhabitants in each of the 395 planning regions. For GPs, 100% coverage is achieved when the ratio of GP to inhabitant reaches 1:1 617. If the coverage of a region exceeds 110%, no further permits are issued (Federal Joint Committee, 2013).

In Denmark, the geographic distribution of physicians is regulated through the access to "provider numbers" in each region (Capital region, Central Jutland, Northern Jutland, Zealand and Southern Denmark). The provider number identifies physicians permitted to be reimbursed by the public tax-based health system. Only these GPs have patients assigned to their lists. The number of provider numbers is set by the regions to guarantee medical service coverage and efficient use of resources. Decisions about provider numbers are based on the number of patients under the gatekeeping scheme (which is the vast majority) in the local area, the individual GP's wish for staff, turnover and list size and the geographical distance of the patient to the practices. The agreed aim is for all patients throughout the country to have a free choice between at least two practices in a 15 km-distance. A GP has the right to close the list if it has reached 1 600 patients. The list is re-opened if the number of patients falls below 1 475 and is closed if it reaches 1 700 patients. Changes in the medical service delivery structure, such as practice relocation, merger with another practice or opening satellite practices, must be in accordance with the regional health plan. If there is a lack of patient capacity within the practices, more provider numbers are issued. The regions can also enter into agreements with GPs to temporarily enlist more patients or to relocate or extend their practice into shortage regions. Since 2011, regions have been allowed to set up their own GP clinics to take care of patients left without a regular doctor, in areas where no qualified physicians are willing to accept a provider number under normal conditions.

Policies targeting international medical graduates

Some countries try to steer physicians into underserved areas by regulating the practice location of international medical graduates (IMGs). These regulations can either attach conditions to immigration for foreign-trained physicians or be part of requirements to obtain full practice rights in the country.

In Australia, a "10-year moratorium" policy on IMGs or "overseas-trained physicians" has been used to tackle a persistent physician shortage in rural and remote locations. The Health Insurance Act Section 19AB restricts IMGs access to Medicare provider numbers, and requires IMGs to work in a district of workforce shortage (DWS) for at least ten years. The aim is to distribute medical services across Australia, and encourage IMGs to work in a DWS to access Medicare benefits by exempting them from the restrictions under Section 19AB.

Physicians can reduce the 10-year period by completing the *Five Year Overseas Trained Doctors Scheme* and work in designated locations where recruitment and retention have been particularly difficult (Australian House of Representatives' Standing Committee on Health and Ageing, 2012). An IMG can also establish a private practice in an eligible location and reduce the ten-year requirement through a "scaling mechanism" depending on remoteness. The growth in GPs (measured in FTE) was 59% in major cities, 42% in regional and 39% in remote areas before the moratorium (between 1984 and 1997). In the period after the moratorium (1997-2011), the growth rates drastically changed with a 20% growth in major cities, 47% in regional and 52% in remote areas

(Cameron and Kosmina, 2013), indicating a relative increase in GP-based rural service provision. In this period, the number of Australian-educated GPs remained broadly constant, while the number of IMGs increased by 240% in major cities, 156% in regional areas and 169% in remote locations.

In Canada, IMGs with no previous North American postgraduate medical training are required to go through a residency programme. A separate matching stream for IMGs for most provinces was established and matching services for clinical training in Canada were managed by the *Canadian Resident Matching Services* (CaRMS, 2010). For IMGs, clinical training in most provinces comes with a return-of-service requirement in an underserved area. They are usually required to provide services for the same duration of time they took to receive their clinical training. Those who do not fulfil the requirement are obliged to repay the full funding with interest. So far no evaluation has been done on this scheme. While it appears effective in placing physicians in the short term, a recent study shows 70% of physicians with a specially funded return-of-service agreement in the province of Newfoundland and Labrador do not fulfil service time or the repayment requirement. One reason for this high default rate is the high proportion of IMGs (74%) who participate in the programme (Mathews et al., 2013).

Depending on their specificities, policies directing IMGs to specific areas could conflict with the WHO Global Code of Practice on the International Recruitment of Health Personnel, adopted by the World Health Assembly in 2010. This voluntary code requires recruiters to give equal treatment and career opportunities to internationally recruited health workers as to those domestically trained (WHO, 2010).

5.7. Doing with less doctors: Service delivery re-orientation

Provider-centred reforms

Provider-centred service re-orientation may comprise fostering group practices of physicians, or of doctors and non-medical health workers, creating networks servicing certain regions and/or introducing new roles. Co-locating services may improve physicians' working conditions by making exchanges with colleagues possible and reducing on-call commitments, and by improving the business case for rural practice as costs may be shared. Another strategy can be sharing responsibilities to serve in certain areas across a network of salaried or self-employed doctors rotating in and out of very remote regions.

Group practices and service co-location

In Germany, 90% of medical students want to work in group practices and community health centres (Hartmannbund, 2012). Results are similar in Canada (Saarma et al., 2012) and Switzerland (Buddeberg-Fischer et al., 2008). Group practices may lead to reduced workload, better resource-sharing and better co-operation with other physicians.

In France, the Maisons de Santé Pluridisciplinaires (MSP) were introduced in 2007. They differ from other forms of group practices because they allow physicians and other health professionals to jointly run group practices while remaining self-employed. MSPs are either entirely financed by the health professionals, or receive subsidies from various sources, such as the European Union, governments and the French health insurance. By 2012, 235 MSPs had been set up in France and another 450 were planned, with 80% of them located in rural areas (Ministère des Affaires sociales et de la Santé, 2012c).

MSPs lead to better work conditions and greater accessibility for patients. In a survey in Franche-Comté and Bourgogne (Bourgueil et al., 2009), 71 GPs in nine MSPs reported a weekly workload of 46 hours compared to 52-60 hours in other practices. MSP opening hours were better with an average of 5.5 opening days/week, and 11.5 opening hours per day. The quality of follow-up care for diabetes patients was also improved.

In Germany, community health centres (MVZ) were established in 2004 through changes to the remuneration scheme of the statutory health insurance system. The aim was to improve physicians' working conditions by reducing their workload, better interaction with other specialties and higher earnings through resource-sharing. MVZ are generally owned by a physician (or groups of physicians) or a hospital and comprise at least two medical specialties. Physicians can be salaried or self-employed. In 2011, there were 1 750 community health centres with a total of 9 571 physicians, mostly GPs and internists. In 2011, 6% of physicians paid by the statutory health insurance worked in MVZ compared to 37% working in other forms of group practice and 57% working in solo practice (KBV, 2011a).

According to a survey by the National Association of Statutory Health Insurance Physicians, 58% of 414 MVZ reported that founding or joining a MVZ was a good decision and 78% said the co-operation among specialties had improved (KBV, 2011b). While 14.6% of MVZs were in rural areas, the rest were in urban areas. Nevertheless, MVZ are considered to hold potential for further expansion in rural areas because the advantages of establishing or joining an MVZ were more pronounced than in urban areas. A 2011 comparison of workload shows that in rural areas, physicians in group practices work on average 4.5 hours less than their colleagues in solo practices, while this difference is only two hours per week in urban areas (Steinhäuser et al., 2011). Work in MVZ in rural regions is also considered economically attractive, as 32% of physicians in rural MVZ reported a strong economic improvement due to resource-sharing compared to 20% in urban areas. Rural MVZ also tend to co-operate more with other medical providers and patients report high degrees of satisfaction (KBV, 2011b).

Network of employed physicians and shared responsibility

In countries where employment rather than self-employment is more common, a network of physicians can support each other. In Japan, most physicians serving isolated rural areas are employed by local government or other public entities and belong in a network providing resources for rural health services. The typical approach to fill vacancies in such areas is a rotation of 2-3 years: if nobody wants to go there permanently, physicians in the region have to share the burden. Patients may not have physicians who know them for their entire life, but they have continued care through the rotation of doctors. Each isolated rural clinic has a corresponding medium-sized hospital providing support for specialist and emergency care. They tend to be a hub of physicians who take turns to rotate so patients may see their previous clinic physicians in a hospital. If it is well organised in a network, continuous care from primary to tertiary care can be provided.

In Scotland, the NHS promoted "obligated networks" in 2009, to improve services through "a formalised arrangement between two or more health care organisations securing access to sustainable services for the whole population served by these organisations". The primary focus is on designated clinical services, ensuring clear pathways of care, visiting service support, and possibly joint staff appointments. A 2010 report cited progress in developing such networks in services such as mental health and learning disabilities (NHS Scotland, 2010).

Introduction or expansion of new provider roles

In areas underserved by doctors, there is potential for role expansion of "mid-level" providers with a more even distribution, such as nurse practitioners or physician assistants. While this is not a new phenomenon (Delamaire and Lafortune, 2010), such roles are increasingly a response to health human resource concerns. Eleven countries indicated in response to the *2012-13 OECD Health System Characteristics Survey* that they had recently introduced such roles or expanded existing roles to provide a larger scope of practice to either address shortages of physicians or relieve the pressures on them (Canada, Chile, Finland, Ireland, the Netherlands, New Zealand, Slovenia, Spain, Sweden, Switzerland and the United States).

In Germany, physicians can delegate home visits of older patients with reduced mobility in rural and remote regions to non-physician practice assistants. These are physician assistants and nurses with an additional qualification designed by the German Medical Association. The services are mostly checking diagnosis-related parameters (such as measuring blood pressure and glucose levels) and basic medical services (such as bandaging and injections). This scheme was implemented nationwide in 2009 by the integration of the remuneration of these services into statutory health insurance. Only services to patients in rural and remote areas aged 65 and above with at least one chronic disease and immobile patients are remunerated (Bundesrat, 2007). The scheme was initiated by the University of Greifswald and tested in Mecklenburg-Western Pomerania, Brandenburg, Saxony and Saxony-Anhalt. At the time of the project evaluation in July 2008, 38 non-physician practice assistants and 53 GPs had participated in the project and 8 386 home visits to 1 486 patients had been undertaken. Out of 42 surveyed GPs, 38 rated the project as "supporting" and "disburdening". Out of 667 patients, 94.3% found that non-physician practice assistants could take over general home visits and 98.7% responded that they were competent service providers.

Processes-centred re-orientation

Fostering the take-up of new processes in health care delivery and involving non-physician care providers in service delivery are ways to ensure access in regions with low physician density.

Support systems/on-call duty management

There is a need to provide short-term cover for absent physicians in underserved regions. This includes cover for permanent staff to have vacation and study leave, but also to enable them to stay in their location without the pressure of being "on call" at all hours. This short-term temporary (locum) cover can be for planned absence (e.g. when the permanent physician is on vacation or study leave) or unplanned absence (e.g. when the permanent doctor becomes ill).

All health services need to arrange cover for absent staff, but the challenges are more pronounced when there may be only one physician in a remote area, or where there are only a few doctors providing a broader range of services in a remote hospital. There is no "on site" ability to co-ordinate cover or provide "on-call" support from other staff because none exist, so cover must be physically brought to the location. If it is a hard-to-fill location, the same factors that make it hard to fill with permanent staff make temporary cover more challenging and often more costly, because of incentives and travel and accommodation costs.

Policy responses to manage the use of locum doctors have been identified in Australia (Skinner et al., 2006), Scotland (Audit Scotland, 2010) and Northern Ireland (Northern Ireland Audit Office, 2011):

- An emphasis on minimising the need to use external locum staff through time planning, work scheduling and co-ordination of study leave and vacation time, and by providing on-call or cross organisational "cross border" support from other permanent staff, where that is feasible.
- Managing locum costs by using in-house co-ordination or by tight cost control of locums.
- Maximising the "fit" between vacancies and locum skills by clear definitions of skill requirements and timely and effective recruitment of locum physicians.
- Developing and implementing organisation-wide standard policies for pre-employment checks, induction, supervision, and performance management of locum physicians.
- Developing appropriate continuous professional development (CPD) requirements reflecting the development needs and requirements of physicians who work long term in locum posts.

Long-term "temporary" staff cover

Some countries use long-term temporary or locum contracts to recruit and retain physicians in "hard-to-fill" locations. These contracts can allow employers to provide additional one-off or recurring incentives such as payments, housing allowances, and end of contract bonuses. This enables additional incentives to small numbers of staff treated as "exceptional" because of the location's challenges. But it has additional cost implications and can raise additional challenges of managing staff on different terms of employment. It may undermine a team ethos if some staff are treated "exceptionally" whilst others are not.

In Australia, outreach Fly-in/Fly-out (FIFO) is used, where mobile doctors and other providers cover large geographic regions on a scheduled or needs-based approach (Health Workforce Australia, 2013a). Physicians living and working in one location are contracted to provide services to remote areas as an adjunct to their primary work (Battye and McTaggart, 2003). A recent report suggested FIFO doctors had helped increase the number of rural general practitioners in regional Western Australia, for the first time since 2008 (ABC News, 2013). These services incur extra costs and require increased management and administrative support to co-ordinate schedules and ensure communities and services are prepared for visits, and necessary follow-up clinical procedures are planned and delivered.

Technology/Telemedicine

The use of technology can reduce the imbalance between rural and urban areas, in terms of service delivery and access. Telemedicine can connect patients and physicians at distance while reducing administrative and travel costs. Technological developments and improved infrastructure enabling telemedicine can be expected to increasingly enter the daily life of physicians' practice.

Whilst telemedicine solutions may provide cost-efficient delivery options in some cases, rural service provision is generally more costly as it often involves a more limited number of patients, meaning smaller economies of scale.

In Canada, a tele-health network in the province of British Columbia began in 2001, using videoconferences to link patients, health-care providers and health-care administrators in 12 communities to resources in Vancouver. It has expanded to approximately 200 tele-health facilities with 470 videoconferencing end points, providing 18 000 consultations in 2007-08 (Ministry of Health of British Columbia). Schaafsma et al. (2007) evaluated a tele-health network with five sites connected with Vancouver. It provides clinical support for maternal/child care, medical, nursing, and health education, and administrative meetings. All sites are equipped with videoconferencing and some also have diagnostic equipment. Annual tele-health use in five sites amounted to 67 clinical consultations, 45 education sessions and 88 administrative sessions. Total travel costs were reduced by CAD 724 457 per year, greater than the annual fixed and variable costs of the telemedicine sessions (CAD 553 740).

5.8. Conclusions

Maldistribution of doctors exists in virtually all OECD countries, in rural and socio-economically disadvantaged regions. Crucial influences on physicians' choice of practice location include the organisation of service delivery, the income potential and working conditions, the prestige and recognition they derive from working in a certain region and specialty, and the origin of doctors.

Three broad strategies are available to respond to imbalances in physician distribution.

- The first is to target future physicians by increasing the number of physicians and/or the number of working hours they provide. The crucial focal point is the selection and type of training provided to medical students.
- The second is to *target current physicians* to maximise those practising in underserved regions.
- The third is to *do with less physicians*, i.e. accept that the number of doctors will be lower in some regions and focus on service re-design or configuration through expanding the involvement of non-physician providers and innovations such as telemedicine.

Policy makers will have to blend strategies, and review this mix over time. The best mix of strategies will depend on patient needs, population and physician demography, health care system characteristics, the budgetary situation, and the overall health reform context.

Table 5.7 provides an overview of possible areas of action, likely impact and cost.

Table 5.7. Strategies, areas of action, impact lag and cost impact to address the uneven geographic distribution of doctors

Strategy	Area of action	Impact lag	Cost structure
Targeting future doctors	Medical education	Long-term	Moderate fixed (upfront) cost, moderate variable cost
Targeting current doctors	Financial incentives	Short to medium term	Significant variable cost
	Regulatory policies	Short term	Moderate variable (administrative) cost
Doing with less physicians	Service delivery reform	Medium to long-term	Significant fixed (upfront) cost, moderate variable cost

In times of austerity, countries may face limitations in what is financially feasible in the short term. This may, by default, orientate policy makers away from options that have upfront cost implications, such as the extension of financial incentives, and towards policy options that are less costly but may take longer to have any impact, such as some education interventions, or may be politically controversial, such as some regulatory changes. It is important that policy makers look beyond the short term when assessing the options. While broad characteristics of interventions can be identified, more robust evaluations are required to improve the evidence base of policies to tackle imbalances in physician supply.

Notes

1. This chapter builds on *OECD Health Working Paper No. 69* (OECD, 2014), providing some data updates and updates in policy responses and evaluations. The authors would like to thank Carol Nader for useful editing.

2. Predominantly urban regions are defined as regions where less than 15% of the population live in rural areas. Predominantly rural regions are defined as regions where more than 50% of the population live in rural areas with no urban centre of at least 200 000 inhabitants accounting for more than 25% of the region's population (OECD, 2011).

References

Aasland, O.G., J.O. Røvik and J. Wiers-Jenssen (2008), "Motives for Choice of Specialty During and After Medical School", *Tidsskr Nor Legeforen*, Vol. 128, pp. 1833-1837.

ABC News (2013), "FIFO Doctors Push Up Regional GP Numbers", Australian Broadcasting Corporation.

Alexandersen, Ø. et al. (2004), "Medisinerutdanningen i Tromsø –sikrer den legerekrutteringen til Nord-Norge?" [Medical education in Tromsø – does it ensure the recruitment of physicians in Northern Norway?], *Tidsskr Nor Lægeforen*, Vol. 16, No. 124, pp. 2107-2109.

AOK Saxony and Thuringia (2011), *Gemeinsame Presseerklärung: Ärzte erhalten finanzielle Förderungen bei Niederlassung in Thüringen* [Joint press declaration: Physicians receive financial support for practice opening in Thuringia].

Audit Scotland (2010), *Using Locum Doctors in Hospitals*, Edinburgh, http://www.audit-scotland.gov.uk.

Australian House of Representatives' Standing Committee on Health and Ageing (2012), *Lost in the Labyrinth: Report on the Inquiry into Registration Processes and Support for Overseas Trained Doctors*, Canberra.

Barlet, M. et al. (2012), "L'accessibilité potentielle localisée (APL) : une nouvelle mesure de l'accessibilité aux médecins généralistes libéraux [Localised potential accessibility: a new measure of accessibility to private GPs] ", *Études et Résultats*, Vol. 795, No. 3, DREES, Paris.

Bärnighausen, T. and D. Bloom (2009), "Financial Incentives for Return of Service in Underserved Areas: A Systematic Review", *BMC Health Services Research*, Vol. 29, No. 9, p. 86.

Battye, K.M. and K. McTaggart (2003), "Development of a Model for Sustainable Delivery of Outreach Allied Health Services to Remote North-west Queensland, Australia", *Rural and Remote Health*, Vol. 3, No. 3, p. 194.

Bennett, K.L. and J.P. Phillips (2010), "Finding, Recruiting, and Sustaining the Future Primary Care Physician Workforce: A New Theoretical Model of Specialty Choice Process", *Acad Med 2010*, Vol. 85(10 Suppl), pp. S81-S88, October.

Bourgueil, Y., J. Mousquès and A. Tajahmadi (2006), "Comment améliorer la répartition géographique des professionnels de santé ? Les enseignements de la littérature internationale et des mesures adoptées en France" [How to improve the geographical distribution of health professionals ? Lessons learned from the international literature and the measures adopted in France], *Rapport No 534*, IRDES, Paris.

Bourgueil, Y. et al. (2009), "An Exploratory Evaluation of Multidisciplinary Primary Care Group Practices in Franche-Comté and Bourgogne", *Issues in health Economics No. 147*, IRDES, Paris.

Buddeberg-Fischer, B. et al. (2008), "The New Generation of Family Physicians – Career Motivation, Life Goals and Work-life Balance", *Swiss Med Weekly 2008*, Vol. 138, No. 21-22, pp. 305-312.

Bundesrat (2007), *Empfehlungen der Ausschüsse, Entwurf eines Gesetzes zur strukturellen Weiterentwicklung der Pflegeversicherung (Pflege-Weiterentwicklungsgesetz)* [Recommendation of the committees, draft law for the structural development of the long-term care insurance (long-term care insurance development law)], *Drucksache 718/1/07*, Berlin.

Cameron, M. and S. Kosmina (2013), "GP Distribution in Rural Australia – Has the OTD Moratorium Worked?", presented at the 12th National Rural Health Conference: Strong Commitment. Bright Future, Adelaide.

Canadian Residency Matching Services (2010), *Canadian Students Studying Medicine Abroad.*

Chandola, T. (2012), "Spatial and Social Determinants of Urban Health in Low-, Middle- and High-income Countries", *Public Health*, Vol. 126, No. 3, pp. 259-226, March.

Cheng, T.C. et al. (2010), "What Factors Influence the Earning of GPs and Medical Specialists in Australia? Evidence from the MABEL Survey", *Melbourne Institute Working Paper Series*, No.12/10, Melbourne Institute of Applied Economic and Social Research.

Colegrove, D.J. and B.E. Whitacre (2009), "Interest in Rural Medicine Among Osteopathic Residents and Medical Students", *Rural and Remote Health*, Vol. 9, No. 1192.

Colorado Health Institute (2012), *A Profile of Colorado's Rural Physicians, Colorado Rural Physician Survey: A Chart Pack*, June 5.

Cooper, J.K., K. Heald and M. Samuels (1972), "The Decision for Rural Practice", *Journal of Medical Education*, Vol. 47, pp. 939-944.

Creed, P.A., J. Searle and M.E. Rogers (2010), "Medical Specialty Prestige and Lifestyle Preferences for Medical Students", *Social Science and Medicine*, Vol. 71, No. 6, pp. 1084-1088, September.

Delamaire, M. and G. Lafortune (2010), "Nurses in Advanced Roles: A Description and Evaluation of Experiences in 12 Developed Countries", *OECD Health Working Papers*, No. 54, OECD Publishing, Paris, http://dx.doi.org/10.1787/5kmbrcfms5g7-en.

Deloitte (2011), *Inntekts- og kostnadsundersokelse for driftsåret 2009 – landets fastleger og avtalespesialister* [Income and cost analysis in 2009 for General practitioners and outpatient specialists], Oslo.

Department of Health and Ageing, Australian Government (2015), *Medical Rural Bonded Scholarship Scheme*, accessed at http://www.health.gov.au/mrbscholarships.

Department of Health and Ageing, Australian Government (2012). *Bonded Medical Places Scheme, Information Booklet for 2013.*

Department of Health and Ageing, Australian Government (2008), *Report on the Audit of Health Workforce in Rural and Regional Australia 2008,* Commonwealth of Australia, Canberra.

Department of Health, Health Service Executive Ireland (2013), *Securing the Future of Smaller Hospitals: A Framework for Development*, Dublin, February.

Dolea, C., L. Stormont and J.-M. Braichet (2010), "Evaluated Strategies to Increase Attraction and Retention of Health Workers in Remote and Rural Areas", *Bull World Health Organ*, Vol. 88, No. 5, pp. 379-385.

Dywili, S. et al. (2012), "Experiences of Overseas Trained Health Professionals in Rural and Remote Areas of Destination Countries – A Literature Review", *Australian Journal of Rural Health,* Vol. 20, pp. 175-184.

Elliott, V.S. (2012), "Who Still Wants To Be a Country Doctor?", *Amed News.*

EU-SILC (2013), *Statistics on Income, Social Inclusion and Living Conditions.*

Federal Joint Committee (2012), *Bedarfsplanungs-Richtlinie* [Planning guideline of the Federal Joint Committee], Federal Ministry of Justice.

Feldman, M.A. et al. (2008), "The Difference Between Medical Students Interested in Rural Family Medicine Versus Urban Family or Specialty Medicine", *Canadian Journal of Rural Medicine*, Vol. 13, No. 2, pp. 73-79, January.

Frehywot. S. et al. (2010), "Compulsory Service Programmes for Recruiting Health Workers in Remote and Rural Areas: Do They Work?", *Bull World Health Organ [online]*, Vol. 88, No. 5, pp. 364-370.

Gibis, B. et al. (2012), "The Career Expectations of Medical Students, Findings of a Nationwide Survey in Germany", *Deutsches Aerzteblatt International*, Vol. 109, No. 18, pp. 327-332.

Greß, S. and K. Stegmüller (2011), *Gesundheitliche Versorgung Stadt und Land, ein Zukunftskonzept* [Health care in cities and the countryside, a future concept], Friedrich Ebert Foundation, Federal Office of Hesse,Wiesbaden.

Grobler, L. et al. (2009), "Interventions for Increasing the Proportion of Health Professionals Practising in Rural and Other Underserved Areas", *Cochrane Database of Systematic Reviews*, Vol. 1, Art. No. CD005314, http://dx.doi.org/10.1002/14651858.CD005314.pub2.

Han, G. and J. Humphreys (2006), "Integration and Retention of International Medical Graduates in Rural Communities: A Typological Analysis", *Journal of Sociology*, Vol. 42, No. 2, pp. 189-207.

Hancock, C. et al. (2009), "Why Doctors Choose Small Towns: A Developmental Model of Rural Physician Recruitment and Retention", *Social Science & Medicine*, Vol. 69, pp. 1368-1376.

Health Workforce Australia (2013) *National Rural and Remote Workforce Innovation and Reform Strategy*, HWA, Adelaide.

Heisler, E.J. (2013), *Physician Supply and the Affordable Care Act*, Congressional Research Service, 15 January.

Henry, L., R.S. Hooker and K.L. Yates (2011), "Role of Physician Assistants in Rural Health Care", *Journal of Rural Health*, Vol. 27, pp. 220-229.

HPM – Harbour Peaks Management Inc. (2008), *British Columbia Rural Physician Programs Review*, March 31.

Huisman, M. et al. (2013), "Socioeconomic Inequalities in Mortality Rates in Old Age in the World Health Organization Europe Region", *Epidemiologic Reviews*, Vol. 35, No. 1, pp. 84-97.

Humphreys, J.S et al. (2008), "Beyond workforce: A Systemic Solution for Health Service Provision in Small Rural and Remote Communities", *Medical Journal of Australia*, Vol. 188, No. 8, p. 77.

IGAS – Inspection générale des affaires sociales (2011), *Pharmacies d'officine : rénumeration, missions* [Community Pharmacy: remuneration, missions], *Réseau*, rapport, Paris.

Inoue, K., M. Matsumoto and T. Sawada (2007), "Evaluation of a Medical School for Rural Doctors", *Journal of Rural Health*, Vol. 23, No. 2, pp. 183-187.

Jakoubovitch, S. et al. (2012), "Les emplois du temps des médecins généralistes" [The timetables of general practitioners], *Études et Résultats*, No. 797, DREES Paris.

Jones, M., J.S. Humphreys and M.R. McGrail (2012), "Why Does a Rural Background Make Medical Students More Likely to Intend to Work in Rural Areas and How Consistent Is the Effect? A Study of the Rural Background Effect", *Australian Journal of Rural Health*, Vol. 20, pp. 29-34.

KBV – National Association of Statutory Health Insurance Physicians (2011a), *Grunddaten zur medizinischen Versorgung in Deutschland* [Basis data on medical service in Germany], Berlin.

KBV (2011b), *MVZ-Survey, Medizinische Versorgungszentren in ländlichen Regionen* [Survey among community health centers, community health centers in rural areas], Berlin.

KBV (2011c), *Beruf und Familie verbinden: Wie sieht das in der Praxis aus?* [Combining work and family: How does this look like in practice?], Berlin.

Laven, G. and D. Wilkinson (2003), "Rural Doctors and Rural Backgrounds: How Strong is the Evidence? A Systematic Review", *Australian Journal of Rural Health*, Vol. 11, No. 6, pp. 277-284.

Lu, D.J., J. Hakes and M. Bai (2008), "Rural Intentions. Factors Affecting the Career Choices of Family Medicine Graduates", *Canadian Family Physician*, Vol. 54, pp. 1016-1017.e1-5.

Mason, J. (2013), *Review of Australian Government Health Workforce Programs,* Department of Health and Ageing, Australian Government.

Mathews, M. et al. (2013), "Evaluation of Physician Return-for-Service Agreements in Newfoundland and Labrador", *Health Care Policy*, Vol. 8, No. 3, pp. 42-53.

Matsumoto, M. et al. (2008), "A Contract-based Training System for Rural Physicians: Follow-up of Jichi Medical University Graduates (1978-2006)", *Journal of Rural Health*, Vol. 24, No. 4, pp. 360-368.

McGrail, M.R. et al. (2012), "How Do Rural GPs' Workloads and Work Activities Differ with Community Size Compared with Metropolitan Practice", *Australian Journal of Primary Health*, Vol. 19, No. 3, pp. 228-233.

McGrail, M.R. et al. (2011), "Nature of Association Between Rural Background and Practice Location: A Comparison of General Practitioners and Specialists", *BMC Health Services Research*, Vol. 11:63.

Ministère des Affaires sociales et de la Santé (2015), *2015 : Pacte territoire santé 2* [Pact territory health 2], 20 November, Paris.

Ministère des Affaires sociales et de la Santé (2012a), *Conclusion des négociations sur la convention pharmaciens d'officine* [Conclusion of negotiations on the convention for pharmacists working in community pharmacies], 29 March, Paris.

Ministère des Affaires sociales et de la Santé (2012b), *Le pacte territoire santé pour lutter contre les déserts médicaux* [The pact territory health to tackle medical desertification], 13 December, Paris.

Ministère des Affaires sociales et de la Santé (2012c), *Les maisons de santé* [Health Homes], Paris.

Ministry of Health of British Columbia (2012), *Rural Retention Program (RRP), Policy Framework for Health Authorities*, June.

Ministry of Health of British Columbia, *Telehealth.*

Natanzon, J. et al. (2010), "Future Potential Country Doctor: The Perspectives of German GPs", *Rural and Remote Health*, Vol. 10:1347.

New York Health (2011), *Health Care Reform in New York City – Access to Primary Health Care before Reform*, Epi Research Report, New York City Department of Health and Mental Hygiene, New York.

NHS Scotland (2010), *Final Report of the Remote and Rural Implementation Group. Remote and Rural Implementation Group*, Edinburgh.

Northern Ireland Audit Office (2011), *The Use of Locum Doctors in Northern Ireland Hospitals*, Belfast.

Northern Ontario School of Medicine (NOSM) (2012), "Distributed Community-engaged Learning", Document prepared for the *Rendez-Vous 2012 Conference*, Thunder Bay, 9-13 October.

OECD (2015), *Health at a Glance 2015: OECD Indicators*, OECD Publishing, Paris, http://dx.doi.org/10.1787/health_glance-2015-en.

OECD (2013), *Regional Database*, available at: http://stats.oecd.org/OECDregionalstatistics/.

OECD (2012), "Gender Equality in Employment", *Closing the Gender Gap: Act Now*, OECD Publishing, Paris, http://dx.doi.org/10.1787/9789264179370-en.

OECD (2011), "Annex A: Territorial Grids and Regional Typology", *OECD Regions at a Glance 2011*, OECD Publishing, Paris, http://dx.doi.org/10.1787/reg_glance-2011-38-en.

OECD (2010), *OECD Rural Policy Reviews: Strategies to Improve Rural Service Delivery,* OECD Publishing, Paris, http://dx.doi.org/10.1787/9789264083967-en.

ONM – Ordre national des médecins (2012), *Observatoire pour la sécurité des médecins, Recensement national des incidents 2012* [Observatory for the security of physicians, National Census of Incidents], Paris.

Ono, T., M. Schoenstein, and J. Buchan (2014), "Geographic Imbalances in Doctor Supply and Policy Responses", *OECD Health Working Papers*, No. 69, OECD Publishing, Paris, http://dx.doi.org/10.1787/5jz5sq5ls1wl-en.

ONP – Ordre national des pharmaciens (2012), *Les pharmaciens – Panorama au 1er janvier 2012* [The pharmacists – Overview in the 1st January 2012], Paris.

PLO – Organisation of General Practitioners in Denmark (2013), *§ 2 aftaler og andre aftaler* [§2-agreements and other agreements], Praktiserende Lægers Organisation.

Rabinowitz, H.K. et al. (2011), "Increasing the Supply of Rural Family Physicians: Recent Outcomes from Jefferson Medical College's Physician Shortage Area Program (PSAP)", *Acad Med.*, Vol. 86, No. 2, pp. 264-269, http://dx.doi.org/10.1097/ACM.0b013e31820469d6.

Regioneres Lønnings- og takstnævn, Praktiserende Lægers Organisation (2011), *Overenkomst om almen praksis* [Agreement on General Practice], 1 April.

Rourke, J. (2010), "How Can Medical Schools Contribute to the Education, Recruitment and Retention of Rural Physicians in their Region?", *Bull World Health Organization*, Vol. 88, pp. 395-396.

Rourke, J. (2008), "Increasing the Number of Rural Physicians", *Canadian Medical Association Journal*, Vol. 178, pp. 322-325.

Rourke, J. (2005), "Strategies to Increase the Enrolment of Students of Rural Origin in Medical School: Recommendations from the Society of Rural Physicians of Canada", *Journal of Ayub Medical* College, Vol. 172, No. 1, pp. 62-65.

Schaafsma, J. et al. (2007), "An Economic Evaluation of a Telehealth Network in British Columbia", *Journal of Telemedicine and Telecare*, Vol. 13, No. 5, pp. 251-256.

Skinner, C. et al. (2006), "The Challenge of Locum Working Arrangements in New South Wales Public Hospitals", *Medical Journal of Australia*, Vol. 185, No. 5,pp. 276-278.

Soethout, M.B.G., G. van der Wal and O.T.J. ten Cate (2007), "Carrierewensen en beroepskeuze van recent afgestudeerden artsen" [Career preferences and choice of a career among recently graduated doctors", *Nederlands Tijdschrift voor Geneeskunde*, Vol. 38, pp. 2118-2124.

URPS Médecins IDF (2013), *Professionnels de santé en Ile-de-France*, basé sur les données de la Caisse autonome de retraite des médecins français de 2009.

Van den Berg, N. et al. (2009), "AGnES: Hausarztunterstützung durch qualifizierte Praxismitarbeiter, Evaluation der Modellprojekte: Qualität und Akzeptanz" [AGnES: GP support by qualified practice assistants, evaluation of model projects: Quality and acceptance], *Deutsches Ärzteblatt International*, Vol. 106, No. 1–2, pp. 3-9.

Van den Hombergh, P. et al. (2005), "Saying 'Goodbye' to Single-handed Practices: What Do Patients and Staff Loose or Gain?", *Family Practice*, Vol. 22, pp. 20-27.

Von Stillfried, D. (2012), "Wirtschafts- und Arbeitssituation der Vertragsärzte – Zielsetzung und Ergebnisse des ZiPP" [Economic situation and working conditions of SHI physicians – goals and results of the Central institute's practice pannel], presentation at conference in Berlin, 20 November 2012.

Weeks, W.B. and A.E. Wallace (2008), "Rural–Urban Differences in Primary Care Physicians' Practice Patterns, Characteristics, and Incomes", *Journal of Rural Health*, Vol. 24, No. 2, pp. 161-170.

Weiskotten, H.G. et al. (1960), "Trends in Medical Practice. An Analysis of the Distribution and Characteristics of Medical College Graduates, 1915-1950", *Journal of Medical Education*, Vol. 35, pp. 1071-1121, December.

WHO (2010), *WHO Global Code of Practice on the International Recruitment of Health Personnel*, World Health Organization, Geneva.

Wilson, N.W. et al. (2009), "A Critical Review of Interventions to Redress the Inequitable Distribution of Healthcare Professionals to Rural and Remote Areas", *Rural and Remote Health*, Vol. 9, No. 2, p. 1060.

Annex 5.A1. Overview of programmes designed to achieve a better geographic distribution of doctors and health services in OECD countries

Table 5.A1.1. Type of programmes to promote a better geographic distribution of doctors and health services in different OECD countries

	Type	Location	Programme	Start year
Medical education policies	Student selection	Australia	Bonded Medical Places Scheme	2004
	Student selection	Australia	Medical Rural Bonded Scholarship	2001 (closed from 2016)
	Student selection	Japan	Regional Quota	2000s
	Medical school for rural area	Norway	Tromsoe Medical School	1972
	Medical school for rural area	Japan	Jichi Medical School	1972
	Regionalised entry into medical education and specialty training	France	*Numerus clausus* policy for entry in medical education Epreuves Classantes Nationales (ECN)	2004
	Distributed medical school in rural area	Canada	Northern Ontario School of Medicine	2005
	Internship	Norway	Finnmark internship programme	1997
	Internship	Australia (NSW)	Rural resident medical officer cadetship programme	1988
	Internships	UK (Scotland)	GP rural fellowships, several medical schools	Varies
Financial incentives	New practice opening incentive	Germany	Financial support for designated shortage	2007
	New practice opening incentive	Canada	Northern and Rural Recruitment and Retention Initiative	2010
	Support for work-life balance	Canada	Financial support to hire locum physicians	At least 2004
	Support for work-life balance	Denmark	Financial support to hire additional staff	2008/2009/2010
	One instalment - retirement	Denmark	Financial incentive for older GPs to postpone retirement	2009/13
	Minimum income guarantee	Denmark	Guaranteed minimum income for two years after practice opening	2008
	Minimum income guarantee	France	Guaranteed minimum income for two years after practice opening	2012
	Bonus for rural practice	Canada	Annual bonus depending on conditions – Rural Retention Programme	2003
	Bonus for rural practice	Denmark	Higher numeration for signing up more patients on the list	2006/07
	Bonus for rural practices	UK (England and Wales)	GP contract renegotiation including rurality index	2004
	Bonus for retirement delay	Canada	Staged annual bonus based on years of practice	2003
	Bonus for retirement delay	Germany	Quarterly support for GPs aged 65 and above	2009
Regulation of practice location	Practice restriction	Germany	No practice permits are issued for overserved areas	1993
	Vacancy determination and practice restriction	Denmark	Practice permits issued based on list size and distance	2011
	Vacancy determination and practice restriction	Norway	Practice permits issued based on list size and general situation in municipality	2001
	Targeting International Medical Graduates	Australia	Ten-year moratorium for access to Medicare payment	1997
	Targeting International Medical Graduates	Canada	Return-of-Service obligation in several provinces	Varies
Service delivery reform	Group practice	France	Maisons de santé pluridisciplinaires	2007
	Group practice	Germany	Medizinisches Versogungszentrum (MVZ)	2004
	Group practice	Switzerland	Financially supported group practices	2007
	Group practice	Japan	Group practice with rotation of multiple clinic	2007
	Group practice/task-sharing	Slovenia	Model practices	2011
	Rotation schemes	UK (Scotland)	Obligated Networks	2009
	Rotation scheme	Ireland	Hospital groups	2013
	Mobile doctors	Australia	FIFO/DIDO programmes	Varies
	Management of on-call duties	AUS/UK (Scotland, Northern Ireland)	Effective management of locum medical staff	Varies
	Telemedicine	Canada	Telemedicine providing clinical support for maternal/child care, education among others	2001
	New roles/task-sharing	Germany	AGnES (non-physician practice assistants) take over GP's home visits	2009
	New roles/task-sharing	France	Pharmacist scope of practice extension	2009

Chapter 6
Skills use and skills mismatch in the health sector: What do we know and what can be done?

By Michael Schoenstein, Tomoko Ono (formerly in OECD Health Division) and Gaetan Lafortune (OECD Health Division)

Health professionals need a wide range of complex skills to perform their work efficiently. However, as in other sectors of the economy, there is not always a perfect match between the skills that health professionals have and the skills required in their jobs. Such skills mismatch raises concerns of a possible waste in human capital (when people are over-skilled for the work they do) or the quality and safety of health services (when they are lacking certain skills). This chapter introduces the concept of skills mismatch among health professionals, proposing a broad framework to analyse both the possibilities of over-skilling and under-skilling. It presents some evidence on the extent of skills mismatch in the health sector by using information reported by doctors and nurses in the 2011-12 OECD Programme for the International Assessment of Adult Competencies (PIAAC) and the 2010 European Working Conditions Survey (EWCS). The results from these two surveys indicate that there tends to be a greater level of skills mismatch among doctors and nurses than among other workers in technical or professional occupations. This chapter then goes on to review some policy levers that might be used to address issues of skills mismatch in the health sector, including policies to expand the scope of practice of certain providers to reduce any over-skilling, and policies related to continuous professional development to ensure that the skills of health care providers remain up-to-date and "fit to practice".

This chapter has been produced with the financial assistance of the European Union. The views expressed herein can in no way be taken to reflect the official opinion of the European Union.

6.1. Introduction

The education and training of health professionals involve substantial investments in time and resources. It takes several years to train new doctors, nurses and other health professionals and their skills need to be kept up-to-date throughout their professional lives. However, as in other sectors of the economy, there is not always a perfect match between the skills of health professionals and their job requirements. Certain health professionals may have acquired more skills than what is required in their job, leading to waste of human capital and job dissatisfaction, whereas others may be lacking some skills to perform certain tasks, possibly leading to lower quality of health services. These different types of skills mismatch generally mean that human resources may be trained and used more efficiently for the sake of improving health care delivery.

While a large body of labour market studies have documented that skills mismatch generally decreases job satisfaction (when people are over-skilled for the work they do), or reduces productivity and quality (when they are under-skilled) (see for instance Quintini, 2011a), relatively few studies have been done on skills mismatch in the health sector, and none that provide a sense of the degree of skills mismatch compared to other sectors. A few studies have examined the extent to which migrant health professionals in particular may be over-qualified or over-skilled because their qualifications may not be recognised in countries where they have moved (e.g. Hussein et al., 2011; van Riemsdijk, 2013). Some other studies have tried to assess the extent of over-skilling among different categories of health care providers, notably nurses, and their possible consequences. For example, findings from the nurse survey under the European RN4CAST project indicate that a very high share of nurses working in hospitals perform tasks that they consider to be below their skill level; immigrant nurses from developing countries in particular consistently report carrying out more tasks below their skill level than domestically-trained nurses (Bruyneel et al., 2013). In a review of Advanced Practice Nurses (APN) in the United States Veterans Administration, Faris and colleagues (2010) found that many APNs were asked to perform basic tasks, negatively impacting their job satisfaction. Furthermore, a qualitative analysis of primary care personnel in the United States Veterans Administration found that many staff were not being used to the extent of their training, and most workers performed many tasks that could reasonably be performed by other personnel with less training (Hysong et al., 2007).

Fewer studies have looked at the impact of skills gaps (under-skilling) on quality and efficiency in health service delivery. Using data from nine of the twelve countries that participated in the European RN4CAST project, Aiken and colleagues (2014) found that a 10% increase in the number of nurses with a bachelor degree education was associated with a 7% decrease in the likelihood of patient mortality in hospital.

The next section (Section 6.2) provides an analytical framework to look at issues of skills mismatch in the health sector, including the definitions of key terms. Section 6.3 reviews some of the evidence on skills mismatch in the health sector, focussing on doctors and nurses in comparison with other technical and professional workers in other sectors, using data from two multi-country surveys: the 2011-12 Programme for the Assessment of Adult Competencies (PIAAC) survey and the 2010 European Working Conditions Survey (EWCS). Section 6.4 then identifies a range of policy levers that might be used to address issues of skills mismatch, either in terms of over-skilling or under-skilling. Section 6.5 concludes.

6.2. Analytical framework

This section presents a framework to analyse skills mismatch in the health sector, including some proposed definitions of key terms.

Labour market studies generally make a distinction between qualifications (and qualifications mismatch) and skills (and skills mismatch). Qualifications generally refer to the acquisition of formal education, diplomas and licenses, whereas skills are defined more broadly as the bundle of knowledge, attributes and capacities that enable people to successfully perform different tasks and can be developed through continuous learning. These skills encompass technical skills as well as a variety of communication, management and other general or specific skills (see Box 6.1, taken from Quintini, 2011).

Figure 6.1 shows that there can be two broad types of skills mismatch in the health sector: 1) *under-skilling* (that is, workers who would benefit from additional training and skills acquisition to better perform some of their tasks); and 2) *over-skilling* (that is, workers who would be able to perform more demanding tasks given their skills level). Such skills mismatches raises three main concerns: 1) *under-skilling* may raise issues about quality and safety in the delivery of health services, if some health workers do not have the skills to perform their duties to the required standards; 2) *over-skilling* means that there is a waste of human capital; and 3) *over-skilling* can also raise issues of job dissatisfaction and turnover (which in turn may reduce quality of care and increase costs).

To minimise concerns about skills mismatches in the health sector, OECD countries regulate tightly the acquisition, certification and use of skills:

- Access to initial education, i.e. the *acquisition of qualifications and skills*, is heavily regulated. Virtually all OECD countries exercise some form of control over who gets to study medicine or nursing, mostly through *numerus clausus* (admission limits) policies. Such control may happen at the beginning of initial education as well as when students enter into post-graduate specialty training for doctors (see Chapter 2).
- The *certification of qualifications and skills* in the health sector is also regulated in all OECD countries. Upon completion of their education, doctors and nurses typically have to pass some form of exam and licensing and registration procedure before they have the right to practise. In addition, several OECD countries (for example, the Czech Republic and Korea) require health professionals, typically doctors, to regularly re-register to ensure that their skills are kept up-to-date.
- The *use of skills* is delineated by regulations defining the scopes of practice of different health occupations in most OECD countries. These may differ from one country to another, but in most countries, certain tasks are clearly associated with a specific occupation due to the required qualification to exercise it. For example, in most OECD countries, only doctors with a medical degree are allowed to prescribe medications. However, some countries have extended to other health professionals, such as Advanced Practice Nurses, the right to prescribe certain medications (Delamaire and Lafortune, 2010).

Figure 6.1. Analytical framework to examine skills mismatch in the health sector

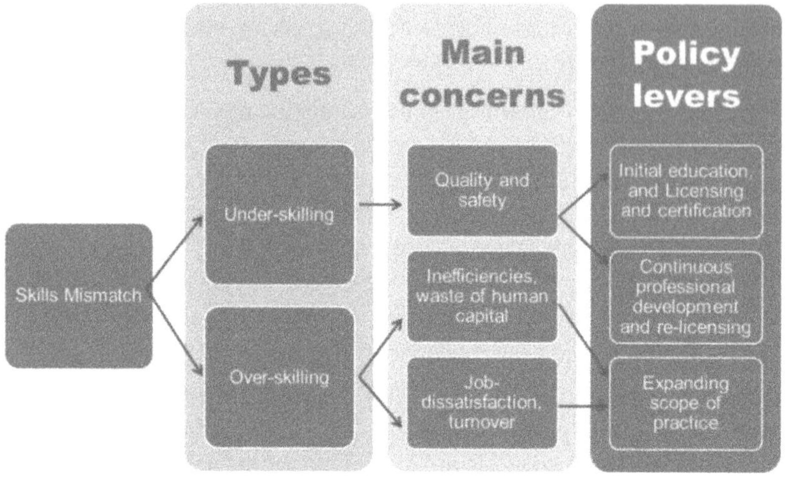

Given the high level of regulation to entry intro medical and nursing professions, one would expect that there would be relatively little *qualification mismatches*, in particular in the form of under-qualified health professionals, as this would violate existing licensing or registration procedures. But *skills mismatches* are more conceivable, given the wide variety and changing nature of skills required in these professions, and that the skills acquired during the education and training periods may not always be used in practice (resulting in over-skilling).

Box 6.1. Glossary of key terms

Qualification mismatch: Discrepancy between the highest qualification held by a worker and the qualification required by his/her job.

Over-qualification: Situation where a worker's highest qualification is higher than the one required by his/her job.

Under-qualification: Situation where a worker's highest qualification is lower than the one required by his/her job.

Skill mismatch: Discrepancy between the skills – both specific and general – possessed by a worker and the skills required by his/her job.

Over-skilling: Situation where a worker's skills are above those required by his/her job.

Under-skilling: Situation where a worker's skills are below those required by his/her job.

Source: Quintini, G. (2011), "Over-qualified or Under-skilled: A Review of Existing Literature", *OECD Social, Employment and Migration Working Papers*, No. 121, OECD Publishing, Paris, http://dx.doi.org/10.1787/5kg58j9d7b6d-en.

6.3. Evidence on skills mismatch in the health sector

One way to shed light on skills mismatch is through analysing data from surveys in which workers are invited to report themselves to what extent their skills match the tasks they perform in their jobs. This section presents findings from two multi-country surveys:

- The 2011-12 wave of the OECD Programme for the International Assessment of Adult Competencies (PIAAC), a comprehensive survey of workers in all sectors of the economy providing information on the use of their skills and skills mismatch. PIAAC allows shifting the focus from traditional proxies of skills, such as years of formal education and training or qualifications/diplomas attained, to a broader perspective that includes the skills people acquire, use and maintain – and also lose – during their lifetime.
- The 2010 wave of the European Working Conditions Survey (EWCS). This survey, launched in 1990 and carried out every five years, aims to measure working conditions in European countries and in its last wave in 2010, included questions related to skills mismatch allowing comparisons of workers in different occupations (Eurofound, 2012).

Table 6.1 provides an overview of the main parameters of these two surveys. Both surveys provide information about how health workers assess their own level of skills mismatch. The EWCS has a relatively small sample size of about 2 000 health workers in 34 countries, including slightly more than 200 doctors and 900 nurses. PIAAC provides information on 5 500 health workers in 22 OECD countries and the Russian Federation, including about 500 doctors and 2 100 nurses. The small sample size in these two surveys limits the level of analysis. To increase the robustness of the results, the data on skills mismatch of doctors and nurses are pooled across all the countries participating in the EWCS and PIAAC surveys. This has the disadvantage of preventing any country-specific analysis.

Table 6.1. Data sources on skills use and skills mismatch

	PIAAC	EWCS
Number of countries	23 Countries	34 countries
Participating countries	Australia, Austria, Belgium, Canada, Czech Republic, Denmark, Estonia, Finland, France, Germany, Ireland, Italy, Japan, Korea, Netherlands, Norway, Poland, Russian Fed., Slovak Republic, Spain, Sweden, United Kingdom and United States	EU28, Norway, The Former Yugoslav Republic of Macedonia, Turkey, Albania, Montenegro and Kosovo
Year	2011-12	2010
Sample size (total)	150 831	43 816
Sample size (health workers/ doctors/nurses)	5 585 / 499 / 2 116	2 093 / 226 / 920
Areas analysed	Qualification mismatch, skills mismatch, skills use	Skills mismatch

Source: OECD (2013), *OECD Skills Outlook 2013: First Results from the Survey of Adult Skills*, OECD Publishing, Paris, http://dx.doi.org/10.1787/9789264204256-en; Eurofound (2012), "Fifth European Working Conditions Survey", Publications Office of the European Union, Luxembourg.

The analysis in this section first presents findings from PIAAC, providing an overview of responses on qualifications mismatch in the health sector before focussing on skills mismatch. The analysis compares the likelihood of respondents indicating any qualifications or skills mismatch to that of workers in other technical and professional occupations (denoted "others"). Then the findings from the EWCS are presented, providing an overview of responses on skills mismatch and an analysis of the likelihood of health workers reporting to be over- or under-skilled.

Findings from PIAAC

This section reviews responses of physicians (doctors) and nurses who participated in the 2011-12 PIAAC survey regarding any qualifications mismatch and skills mismatch.

Qualifications mismatch is low

As already noted, the high level of regulation concerning the education and training of health professionals, and the certification of their skills when they enter the profession through licensing and registration requirements, implies that there should be little (if any) mismatch between their initial qualifications and their jobs.

Figure 6.2 confirms this by showing that a higher percentage of doctors and nurses reported that they have the right qualifications for their jobs, compared with workers in other technical and professional occupations (denoted "others"). While almost a quarter of workers in other technical and professional occupations indicated a mismatch between their qualifications and their jobs, 89% of doctors indicated that their qualification matched their job. Only 4% indicated that their job could be fulfilled with a lower qualification, while 7% indicated they would need a higher qualification. The percentage of a good qualification match is slightly lower for nurses, with 81% reporting they have the right qualifications for their job, while 10% said they are over-qualified and the remaining 9% said they are under-qualified for the job they are doing.

Figure 6.2. Low qualifications mismatch reported among health professionals compared to other workers, pooled data from 21 countries participating in the PIAAC survey, 2011-12

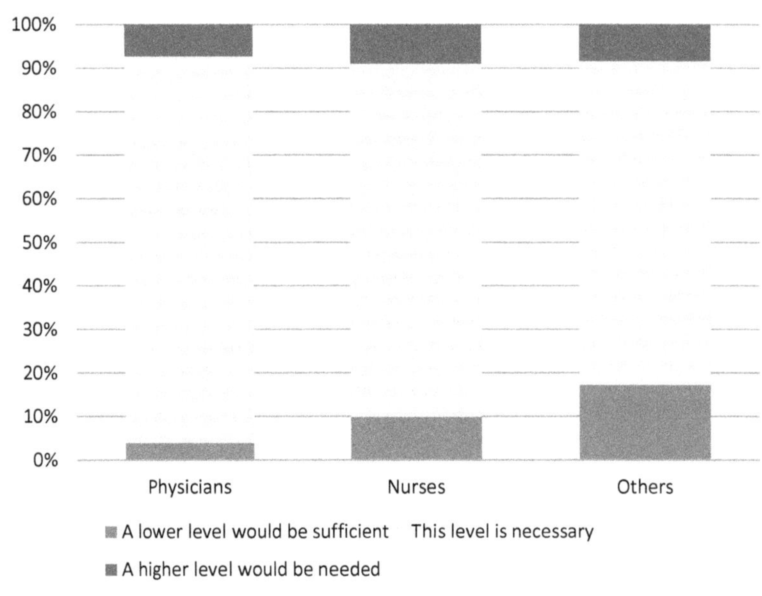

Note: "Others" refers to workers in other technical and professional occupations (ISCO 2 and 3).

Source: PIAAC, OECD analysis.

StatLink http://dx.doi.org/10.1787/888933326480

Many physicians and nurses report being over-skilled, but less so than workers in other occupations

Figure 6.3 shows that more than three-quarters of physicians and nurses who responded to the PIAAC survey reported being over-skilled, but still a slightly lower proportion than workers in other technical and professional occupations. To be precise, 76% of doctors and 79% of nurses reported they had the skills to cope with more demanding tasks in their jobs. This was slightly smaller than the average of 84% for workers in other technical and professional occupations. It is important to note that the survey allows for respondents to simultaneously indicate that they are over-skilled for some parts of their work and under-skilled for some other parts.

Figure 6.3. Reported over-skilling by physicians, nurses and other occupations, PIAAC Survey, 2011-12

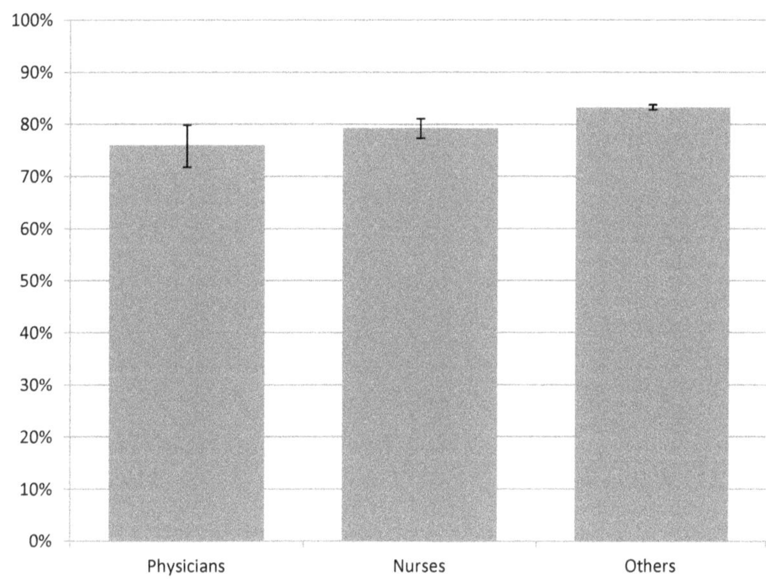

Note: Others = workers in other technical and professional occupations (ISCO 2 and 3). The figure depicts percentage responses with the associated 95% confidence interval.

Source: PIAAC, OECD analysis.

StatLink http://dx.doi.org/10.1787/888933326492

Results from the RN4CAST project in relation to nurses are broadly consistent with the levels of over-skilling reported in PIAAC. The RN4CAST nurse survey covered about 33 000 nurses working in 486 hospitals in 12 EU countries (Belgium, Finland, Germany, Greece, Ireland, Norway, Poland, Spain, Sweden, Switzerland, the Netherlands and England). The survey collected information on the share of nurses who reported performing tasks below their skill level, including tasks such as delivering and retrieving food trays, transporting patients within the hospital, cleaning patient rooms and equipment, and obtaining supplies or equipment. In every country, at least three of the nine tasks deemed to be below their skill level were carried out by at least 70% of nurses who responded to the survey (Bruyneel, 2013).

Higher proportions of doctors and nurses reporting to be under-skilled than workers in other technical and professional occupations

Among doctors who responded to the PIAAC survey, slightly more than half (51%) reported they felt they would need further training to cope well with their present duties. Among nurses, the share of respondents reporting such under-skilling was 43%. This level was not significantly statistically different from the average of 40% of workers in other technical and professional occupations (Figure 6.4).

Figure 6.4. Reported under-skilling by physicians, nurses and other occupations, PIAAC Survey, 2011-12

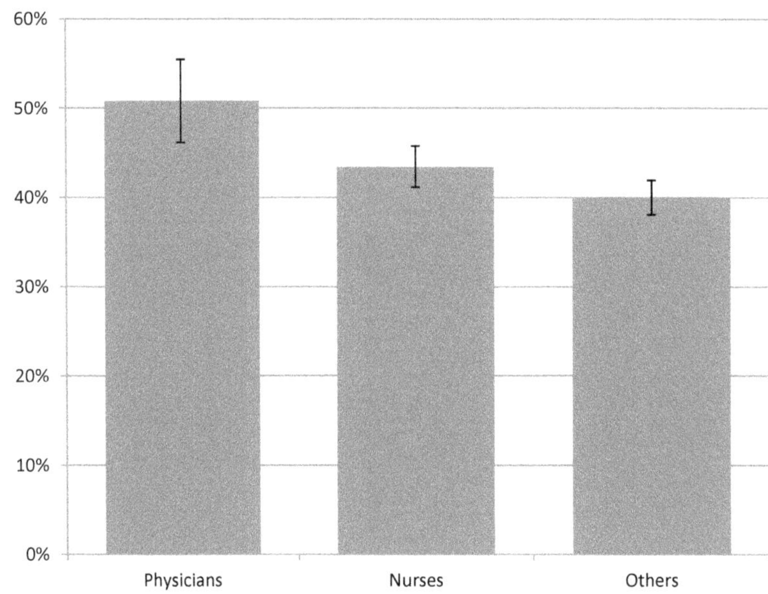

Note: Others = workers in other technical and professional occupations (ISCO 2 and 3). The figure depicts percentage responses with the associated 95% confidence interval.

Source: PIAAC, OECD analysis.

StatLink http://dx.doi.org/10.1787/888933326509

It is not possible to find out from PIAAC which specific skills those health professionals who reported to be under-skilled considered they were lacking. It is not known whether this relates, for example, to administration and management skills, IT (computer) skills or clinical skills. Therefore, such self-reports of under-skilling do not necessarily mean that health professionals are not capable of fulfilling their clinical duties. It means simply that for some aspects of their work, they feel they would need more training to cope better with their duties.

However, PIAAC contains information about the extent to which workers use different skills in their jobs which helps to contextualise responses about under-skilling. Skills are grouped into five major categories: 1) problem-solving skills, 2) self-organising skills, 3) co-operative skills, 4) dexterity, and 5) physical skills. Doctors and nurses generally indicated that they frequently use a more diverse set of skills than workers in other technical and professional occupations, making their jobs more complex.

Among doctors, the share of respondents indicating that they use these skills every day or at least once a week was higher than the percentage of workers in other technical and professional occupations for each of these five categories of skills. Among nurses, the percentage reporting to use problem-solving skills at least once a week or every day was lower than for other professionals, but the share of nurses using co-operative, self-organising, physical skills, or dexterity was higher than that of workers in other technical and professional occupations (Figure 6.5).

Figure 6.5. Reported skills use by physicians, nurses and other occupations, PIAAC, 2011-12

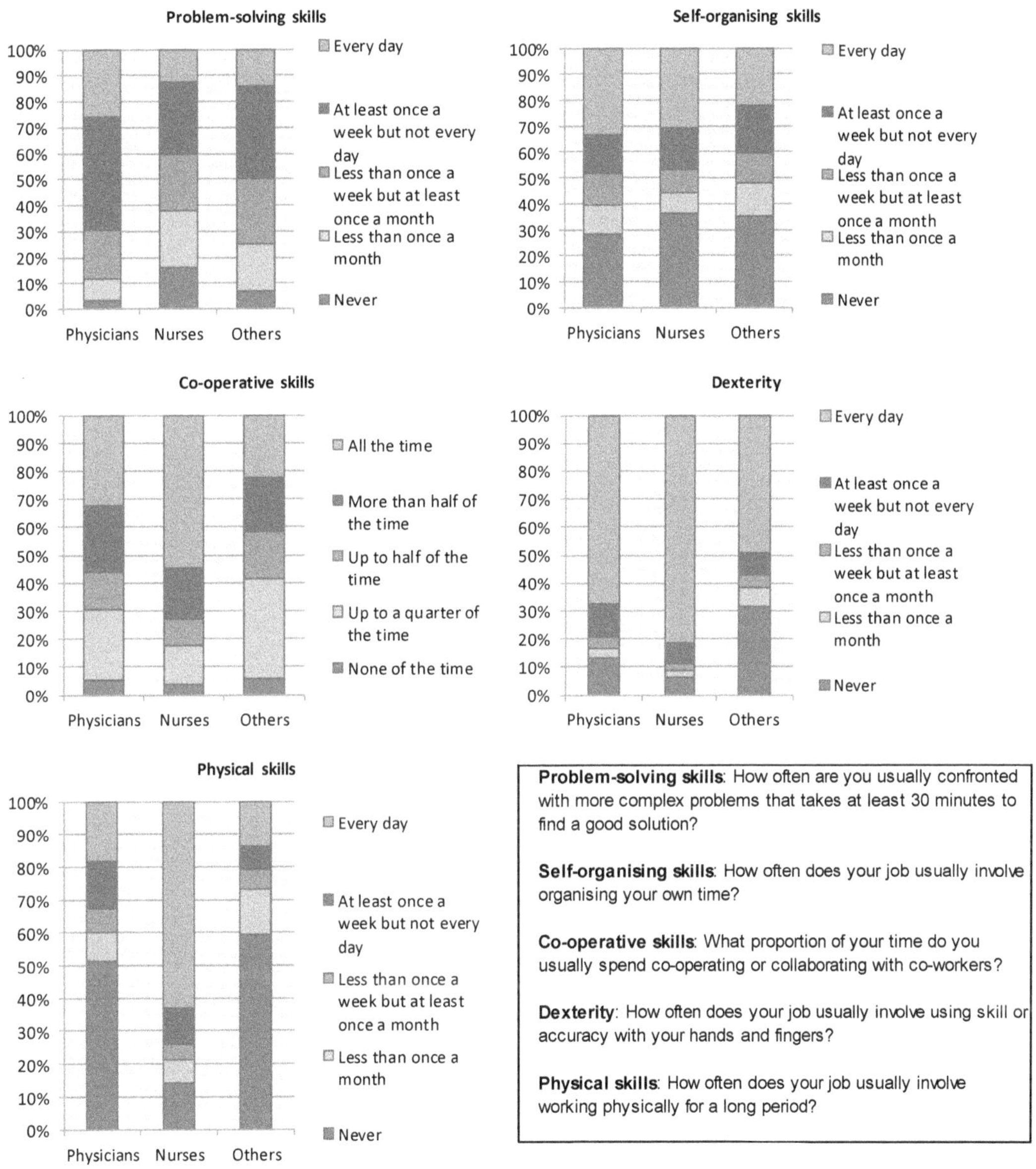

Source: PIAAC.

StatLink http://dx.doi.org/10.1787/888933326512

Likelihood of reporting being over-skilled or under-skilled

This section presents the results from the PIAAC survey in terms of the likelihood of a respondent indicating being over- or under-skilled, while taking into account differences in the age and gender composition of the doctors and nurses as well as adjusting for possible country-specific biases.

Figure 6.6 confirms the gradient of responses previously shown from that survey. Both doctors and nurses were slightly less likely to report being over-skilled, and more likely to report being under-skilled, than workers in other technical and professional occupations, after adjustments for differences in the age and gender composition of the different occupations. Doctors were 46% less likely to report being over-skilled than workers in other technical and professional occupations, while this proportion was 16% for nurses. On the other hand, doctors were 67% more likely, and nurses 14% more likely, to report being under-skilled than workers in other technical and professional occupations (denoted "other workers").

Figure 6.6. Likelihood of reporting being over-skilled or under-skilled by occupation in PIAAC, 2011-12

Multinomial logistic regression, odds ratios

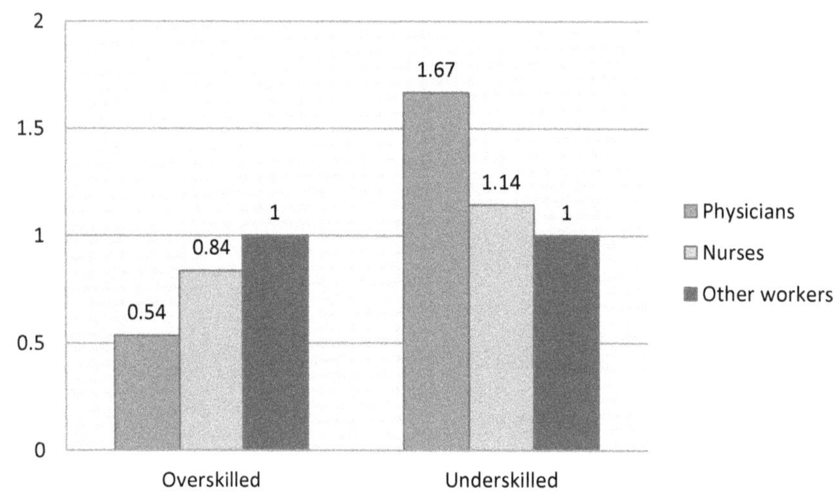

Note: "Others" refers to workers in other technical and professional occupations (ISCO 2 and 3).

Source: PIAAC data, OECD analysis.

StatLink http://dx.doi.org/10.1787/888933326529

Findings from the EWCS

The European Working Conditions Survey (EWCS) covers a different set of countries (see Table 6.1) and differs from the PIAAC survey in the structure of questions related to skills mismatch. Respondents to the EWCS survey cannot indicate *simultaneously* whether they might be over- and under-skilled for different tasks in their job. Rather, they are asked for an overall assessment of whether their skills generally match the requirements for their job. As a consequence, the percentages of respondents reporting to be either over-skilled or under-skilled are significantly lower than in the PIAAC survey.

Figure 6.7 shows that:

- 27% of doctors and 28% of nurses reported being over-skilled in the 2010 EWCS survey, a slightly lower proportion compared with the average of workers in other technical and professional occupations (30%).
- 25% of doctors reported being under-skilled, compared with 17% of nurses, and 17% also of workers in other technical and professional occupations.
- Taken together, this means that only 48% of doctors and 55% of nurses felt that, overall, they had the right skills to do their work. The proportion for nurses was comparable to that of workers in other technical and professional occupations (Figure 6.7).

Figure 6.7. Reported skills mismatch by physicians, nurses and other occupations, EWCS survey, 2010

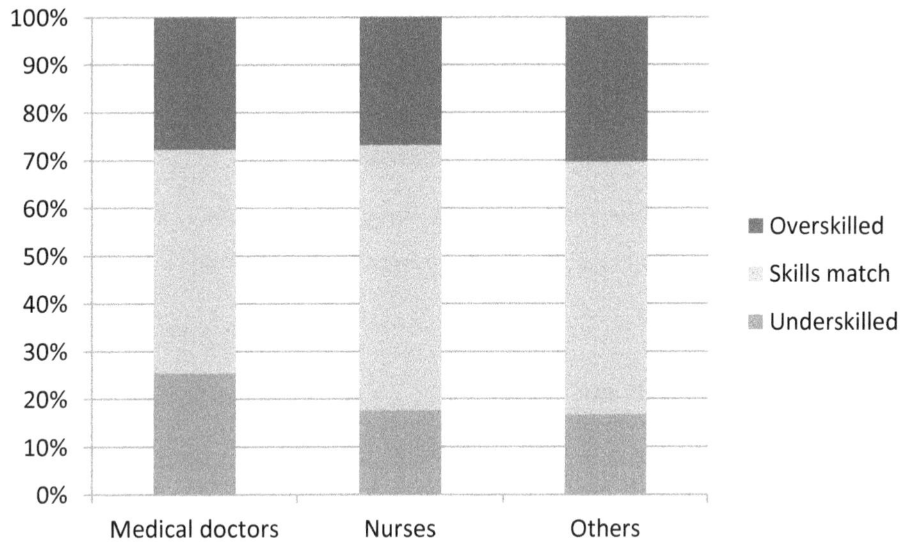

Note: "Others" refers to workers in other technical and professional occupations (ISCO 2 and 3)

Source: EWCS (Eurofound, 2012, "Fifth European Working Conditions Survey", Publications Office of the European Union, Luxembourg).

StatLink http://dx.doi.org/10.1787/888933326535

When adjusting for differences in the age and sex composition of different occupational groups, there is little difference in the likelihood of doctors and nurses reporting to be over-skilled compared to workers in other technical and professional occupations. For doctors, the likelihood is 2% higher, while for nurses it is 8% lower than for workers in other occupations.

The likelihood that doctors consider themselves to be under-skilled is, however, 82% higher than for workers in other technical and professional occupations, while for nurses it is 6% higher (Figure 6.8). These results are very similar in terms of gradient to those found from the statistical analysis of PIAAC responses in that the likelihood of over-skilling appears to be much less pronounced than that of under-skilling.

Figure 6.8. Likelihood to report being over-skilled or under-skilled by occupation (adjusted by age and sex of different occupations), EWCS survey, 2010

Multinomial logistic regression, odds ratios

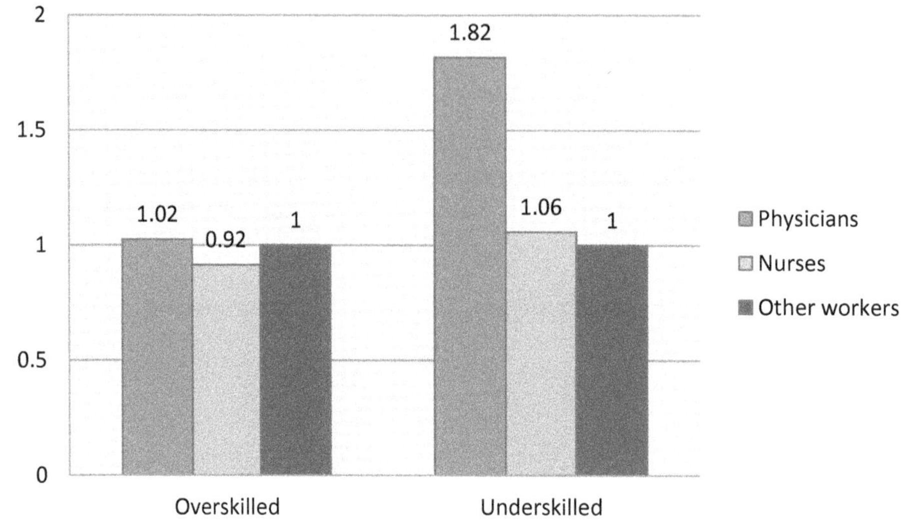

Note: "Other workers" refers to workers in other technical and professional occupations (ISCO 2 and 3)

Source: EWCS (Eurofound, 2012, "Fifth European Working Conditions Survey", Publications Office of the European Union, Luxembourg). OECD analysis.

StatLink http://dx.doi.org/10.1787/888933326540

6.4. Policy levers to address skills mismatch

This section discusses some possible policy levers that might be used to address any skills mismatch among health professionals, with a continued focus mainly on doctors and nurses. Addressing any over-skilling or under-skilling issues is important to make sure that there is a good return on the large investments that are made in the education and training of health professionals and to promote quality of care and patient safety.

A crucial policy lever to make sure that future generations of doctors and nurses will have the right skills to be "fit for practice" relates to the design of initial medical and nursing education programmes, since it is during these formative years that they will acquire a large part of the skills that they will use throughout their professional lives. A *Lancet* Commission on the training of health professionals for the 21st century called for more attention to problem-based learning and team-based training of different health professionals to overcome current gaps between the skills acquired in schools and the requirements in the workplaces and improve the distribution of tasks across the spectrum of health professions (Frenk et al., 2010). Problem-based learning can be described as a learning environment where the problem drives the teaching, and knowledge and skills are acquired in a context that is as close as possible to where it will be applied later in practice. Greater problem-based learning has been effective not only in improving the problem-solving skills of students, but also in improving their social and communication skills (Klegeris and Hurren, 2011; Skochelak, 2010).

This section does not focus on these important issues related to the design of initial education programmes for doctors and nurses. Rather, it focusses on policies to address any skills mismatch among currently practicing health workers, with a particular focus on policies to extend the scope of practice of certain "mid-level" health care providers (e.g., advanced practice nurses) and to promote the continuous professional development of doctors and nurses for regular skills updating.

Policies to address issues of over-skilling: Extension of scope of practice of "mid-level" providers

Several OECD countries are addressing issues of the over-skilling of doctors and nurses for certain tasks by extending the scope of practice of certain providers and/or introducing new roles, often with the aim of improving access to primary care for the whole population. According to information collected through the *2012-13 OECD Health System Characteristics Survey*, about half of OECD countries have introduced or expanded the roles of non-physicians between 2007 and 2012 (Table 6.2). Although in Chile introduction or expansion of non-physicians roles concerned midwifes or ophthalmologists, across OECD countries, this has often involved expanding the number and roles of advanced practice nurses, such as nurse practitioners.

Table 6.2. Recent introduction or expansion of non-physician provider roles, OECD countries, 2012-13

Recent introduction or expansion of non-physician provider roles (over past five years)	No introduction or expansion of non-physician roles
Australia	Austria
Canada	Belgium
Chile	Czech Republic
Finland	Germany
France	Greece
Denmark	Hungary
Ireland	Iceland
Netherlands	Israel
New Zealand	Italy
Norway	Japan
Slovenia	Korea
Spain	Luxembourg
Sweden	Mexico
Switzerland	Poland
United Kingdom	Portugal
United States	

Source: 2012-13 OECD Health System Characteristics Survey.

Previous OECD work has shown that the development of new nursing roles varies greatly across OECD countries. The United States and Canada established nurse practitioners all the way back to the mid-1960s in an effort to improve access to primary care to populations living in rural and remote areas where very few doctors were practicing, and their numbers have continued to grow in recent years (see Chapter 2). Other Anglo-saxon countries such as the United Kingdom, Ireland and Australia also have a long experience in training and using nurse practitioners to perform certain clinical tasks that were previously performed solely by doctors. In most countries, a graduate degree in nursing (often a master's degree) is normally required to qualify as a nurse practitioner, although there are some exceptions where a bachelor's degree may still be sufficient to enter into these "mid-level" occupations (Delamaire and Lafortune, 2010).

Evaluations of experiences with nurse practitioners and other advanced practice nurses show that they can improve access to services and reduce waiting times. Nurse practitioners are able to deliver the same quality of care as doctors for a range of patients, including those with minor illnesses and those requiring routine follow-up, when they have received proper education and training. Most evaluations find a high patient satisfaction rate, mainly because nurses tend to spend more time with patients, and provide information and counselling (Delamaire and Lafortune, 2010).

In many countries, there remain however significant barriers to the introduction or expansion of the scope of practice for non-physicians, such as advanced practice nurses. The involvement of stakeholder groups in reform discussions is crucial, as the position of professional associations – in particular medical associations and nurse associations – plays an important role in determining the possibility and speed of implementation of new roles. The organisation and financing of health care is another crucial factor in determining the extent to which the scope of practice roles may grow. For example, the introduction of nurse practitioner roles outside hospitals may be more difficult where doctors operate mainly in private solo practices and paid fee-for-services, and easier where there are more group practices.

A major challenge in introducing new roles is effective co-ordination between employers and training institutions. Employers require changes to legislation and regulation to remove barriers to extending the scopes of practice of some of their workers, and re-organisation of care to involve them efficiently in the provision of health services. It is crucial to ensure that there are a sufficient number of posts that can absorb nurses who wish to practise at a higher level and have the qualifications and skills to do so, or else they will be over-qualified and over-skilled if they have to take more traditional nursing positions. In France, discussions continue on the possible recognition of a nurse practitioner role in primary care, although some advance practice nursing roles have been recognised now in certain areas like cancer care and training programmes at the master's level have been created to fill these posts.

Figure 6.9 shows an analysis of nurses responses to PIAAC, comparing the likelihood of nurses with a degree lower than bachelor's level (n=155) to report being over- or under-skilled with nurses who have a bachelor's degree or equivalent (n=567) and those with a master's degree (n=478), adjusting for age. As expected, nurses with higher degrees are more likely to indicate being over-skilled and less likely to be under-skilled than those with lower degrees. Nurses with a master's degree were 66% more likely to report being over-skilled than those without a bachelor's degree and over 80% more likely to report being over-skilled compared with those with a bachelor's degree. This indicates that there is a substantial under-utilisation of the more advanced skills that these highly educated nurses have acquired in many countries.

Figure 6.9. Skills mismatch among nurses by level of education, PIAAC, 2011-12

Multinomial logistic regression, odds ratios

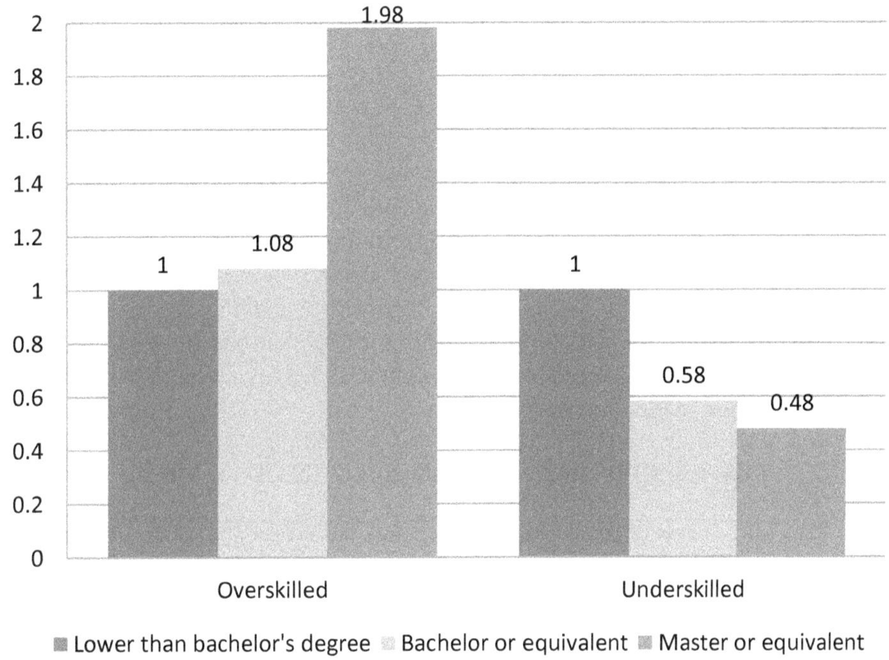

Source: PIAAC, OECD analysis.

StatLink http://dx.doi.org/10.1787/888933326550

In the United Kingdom, the introduction of new roles in health care is supported by a sector-specific skills council, *UK Skills for Health*. This Council, which is funded publicly, is designed to foster health workforce innovation through raising employer engagement, demand and investment in skills, developing national occupational standards and ensuring qualifications meet employer needs. Since its inception in 2002, *Skills for Health* has helped employers at a local level to transform emerging practice patterns into formalised new roles, along with designing appropriate training opportunities. At the same time, it has helped to scale successful new roles at a national level. According to an evaluation by the UK National Audit Office, the work of the Skills Council has led to significant cost savings, through for example the introduction of a new emergency care practitioner role developed in partnership with stakeholders (National Audit Office, 2009).

Policy levers to address issues of under-skilling: Continuous professional development

Continuous professional development (CPD) is one the main policy levers to ensure that the skills of doctors and nurses currently in practice are kept up-to-date in a context of changing technologies and job requirements. Increasingly, participation in CPD activities is combined with re-licensing or re-registration requirements, as part of important health workforce management processes to ensure quality and patient safety. There is growing recognition that awarding a license to practise at the end of medical or nursing education is not sufficient to ensure high quality of care throughout the whole career span, particularly considering the rapidly changing nature of health care delivery.

Policies and regulations concerning CPD vary greatly across OECD countries. There are variations notably regarding whether participation in CPD activities is mandatory or not, whether there are requirements for health professionals to renew their licenses or registrations, and where that is the case, whether a certain amount of CPD is a mandatory part of the re-licensing or re-registration process.

Table 6.3 illustrates the diversity of policy and regulatory approaches concerning CPD for doctors, based on responses to the *2012-13 OECD Health System Characteristics Survey*. Out of the 31 OECD countries which responded to these survey questions, nine countries indicated that they had no formal system of CPD for doctors, but this does not mean that there is no training requirement in place. Nineteen countries indicated that a formal system of CPD for doctors was in place, and in a majority of them that CPD was mandatory. Only 12 countries reported that CPD for doctors was both mandatory and linked to re-licensing. In the United Kingdom, CPD is linked to re-licensing or re-registration protocols, although CPD provisions for doctors do not follow a uniform nation-wide system.

Table 6.3. CPD regulation for doctors in OECD countries

No formal CPD system for doctors	Formal CPD system for doctors	For all doctors (all specialties)	Mandatory and linked to re-licensing	Mandatory but not linked to re-licensing
Australia	X	x	x	
Austria	X	x		x
Belgium	X	x	x	
Canada	X	x		x
Chile				
Czech Republic	X	x	x	
Denmark				
Finland				
France	X	x		
Germany	X	x		x
Greece				
Hungary	X	x	x	
Iceland				
Ireland	X	x	x	
Israel	X	-		
Italy	X	x		x
Japan	X	x		
Korea	X	x	x	
Luxembourg				
Mexico				
Netherlands	X	x	x	
New Zealand	X	x	x	
Norway	X		x	
Poland	X	x		x
Portugal				
Slovenia	X	x	x	
Spain	X	x		x
Sweden				
Switzerland	X	x		x
United Kingdom			x	

Source: OECD Health Systems Characteristics Survey 2012-13.

A wide range of CPD activities may be available to doctors and nurses, but the most popular according to the results from the 2011-12 PIAAC survey are participation in seminars and workshops for doctors, and some form of on-the-job training for nurses (Figure 6.10). Open or distance learning (E-learning) are less common, although one-in-four doctors and one-in-six nurses reported participating in an open or distance learning in the previous year (Figure 6.10).

Figure 6.10. Reported training experience in the past 12 months, by type of training and occupation, PIAAC, 2011-12

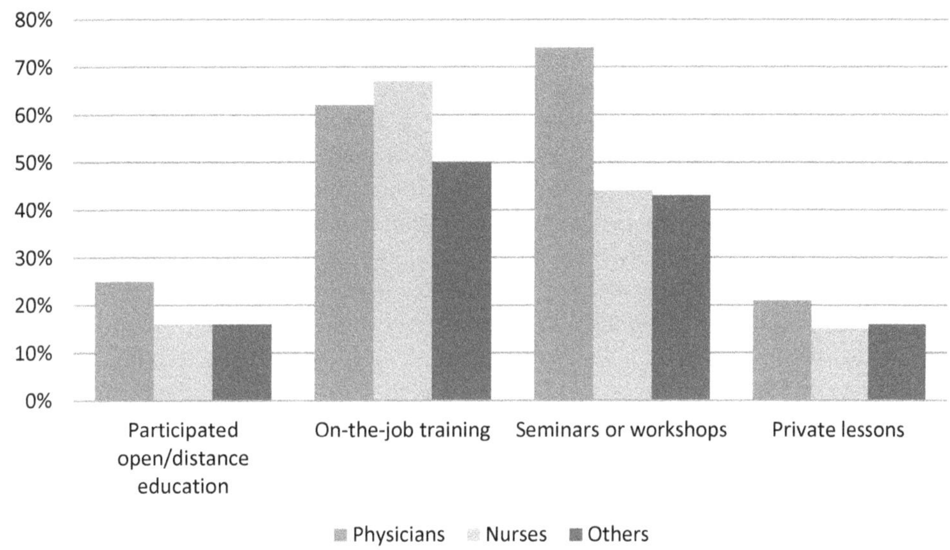

Note: "Others" refers to workers in other technical and professional occupations (ISCO 2 and 3).

Source: PIAAC.

StatLink http://dx.doi.org/10.1787/888933326564

At the European level, a recent study described CPD models, approaches and practices across all EU countries and EFTA countries for five health professions: doctors, nurses, dentists, midwives and pharmacists. This study confirmed that CPD systems vary widely both across professional groups and across countries in Europe, with some countries having mandatory systems sometimes related to re-licensing/re-registration across some or all professions while others are based more on voluntary participation (European Commission, 2014).

Regardless of whether mandatory or voluntary systems are in place this European study identified some key common barriers to greater participation in CPD activities for doctors, nurses and other health professionals, namely lack of time and related cost. One of the main recommendations of this study was to consider CPD as a shared responsibility between employers, professional organisations and ministries of health, along with the health professionals themselves, and that there was a need for more systematic and organisational support to allow professionals to take time off for CPD and to ensure that the costs are not prohibitive. This study also recommended to make use of flexible learning tools and to ensure that CPD is relevant to the daily practice of health professionals to improve access and perceived benefits (European Commission, 2014).

A common issue in CPD systems is to find out more about the specific training needs of different health professionals, based on self-reports and on achieving certain standards, and to respond to these needs in the most efficient way. Data from currently available national or international surveys, such as PIAAC and EWCS, are not really suited to provide such specific information about skills gaps and training needs.

6.5. Conclusions

The analysis presented in this chapter shows that health professionals have a low degree of qualification mismatch compared with workers in other technical and professional occupations. Licensing and registration requirements appear effective in matching qualifications to jobs in the health sector.

However, the available evidence from two multi-country surveys – PIAAC and the EWCS – indicate that even if there is a good match in initial qualifications, doctors and nurses themselves report a certain degree of skills mismatch, as some report being over-skilled for certain tasks they have to do on the job and others report being under-skilled (i.e., lacking skills) for certain tasks. Among respondents from the 22 OECD countries that participated in the PIAAC survey in 2011-12, doctors and nurses were less likely to report being over-skilled than workers in other technical and professional occupations, while a greater proportion of doctors and nurses reported being under-skilled. However, among nurses, those with a high level of education (e.g., a master's degree) were much more likely to report being over-skilled, and much less likely to report being under-skilled, than those with a lower level of education. Among respondents from the 34 European countries included in the 2010 wave of the EWCS survey, doctors and nurses were equally as likely to report being over-skilled compared with workers in other technical and professional occupations, while doctors were more likely to report being under-skilled for certain tasks (which was not the case for nurses).

Taken together, these findings suggest that there is a considerable level of skills mismatch among doctors (and to a lesser extent among nurses), greater than for other technical and professional occupations. The different types of skills mismatch raise different issues: while doctors and nurses who report being over-skilled for the work they do raise concerns about a waste of human capital (given that education and training is expensive) and often generates considerable job dissatisfaction, those who report being under-skilled raise other issues regarding the quality and safety of services provided. Achieving a better match between the skills that people have and their job requirements may therefore help achieve efficiency gains and quality gains.

The issue of skills mismatch raises questions not only about the initial education of doctors and nurses – a crucial period of course in terms of skills acquisition – but also about what happens to doctors and nurses once they have completed their initial medical and nursing degree in terms of their work practice and opportunities for continuous professional development and lifelong learning.

Based on the results from the *2012-13 OECD Health System Characteristics Survey*, about half of OECD countries reported having taken steps in recent years to either introduce or expand the scopes of practice for certain non-physician providers such as advanced practice nurses, to allow them to use their skills more fully and to free up time for doctors to focus on more complex tasks and patients. As the education and training of such advanced practice nurses and other "mid-level" providers increases in many countries, it will be important to ensure that there will be sufficient opportunities for them to use their skills in the workplace after graduation.

It is also critical to promote continuous professional development of doctors and nurses after they have graduated, so that their skills remain up-to-date. There continue to be lively debates in many countries about the best policies and approaches to promote continuous professional development, and whether it should be made mandatory and linked to re-licensing and re-certification. While many countries have adopted this approach for some or all regulated health professionals, others have chosen a more voluntary approach. There is are also a need to reduce barriers to CPD participation by making sure that health professionals have a certain amount of time dedicated to these activities, that the cost is affordable, and that the CPD programmes are properly designed and relevant in improving their daily practice.

Available data sources at the national and international level to measure any skill gaps among health professional remain too general, limited in scope, and with too small sample sizes seriously limiting the possibility to analyse the information by profession, age and gender. Given the large amount of money already spent in the education and training of health professionals, there is a need to invest a certain amount of resources to identify more clearly the skills requirements and skills mismatches. A more careful assessment of skills mismatches should play a more central role in health workforce management.

References

Aiken, L. et al. (2014), "Nurse Staffing and Education and Hospital Mortality in Nine European Countries: A Retrospective Observational Study", *The Lancet*, published online 26 February.

Aiken, L. et al. for the RN4CAST Consortium (2013), "Nurses' Reports of Working Conditions and Hospital Quality of Care in 12 Countries in Europe", *International Journal of Nursing Studies*, Vol. 50, No. 2, pp. 143-153, February.

Aiken, L. et al. (2012), "Patient Safety, Satisfaction, and Quality of Hospital Care: Cross Sectional Surveys of Nurses and Patients in 12 Countries in Europe and the United States", *British Medical Journal*, Vol. 344, p. e1717, published online 20 March.

Bruyneel, L. et al. (2013), "A Multi-country Perspective on Nurses' Tasks Below Their Skill Level: Reports from Domestically Trained Nurses and Foreign Trained Nurses from Developing Countries", *International Journal of Nursing Studies*, Vol. 50, No. 2, pp. 202-209, February.

Delamaire, M. and G. Lafortune (2010), "Nurses in Advanced Roles: A Description and Evaluation of Experiences in 12 Developed Countries", *OECD Health Working Papers*, No. 54, OECD Publishing, Paris, http://dx.doi.org/10.1787/5kmbrcfms5g7-en.

Dubois, C.A. and D. Singh (2009), "From Staff-mix to Skill-mix and Beyond: Towards a Systemic Approach to Health Workforce Management, Human Resources for Health", Vol. 7, No. 87, published online December 19.

Eurofound (2012), "Fifth European Working Conditions Survey", Publications Office of the European Union, Luxembourg.

European Commission (2014), *Study Concerning the Review and Mapping of Continuous Professional Development and Lifelong Learning for Health Professionals in the EU – Final Report*, funded by the European Union in the frame of the EU Health Programme 2008-103, EAHC/2013/Health/07.

Faris, J.A. et al. (2010), "Job Satisfaction of Advanced Practice Nurses in the Veterans Health Administration", *Journal of the American Association of Nurse Practitioners*, Vol. 22, No. 1, pp. 35-44, January.

Frenk, J. et al. (2010), "Health Professionals for a New Century: Transforming Education to Strengthen Health Systems in an Interdependent World", *The Lancet*, Vol. 376, pp. 1923–1958.

Gilles, I., B. Burnand and I. Peytremann-Bridevaux (2014), "Factors Associated with Healthcare Professionals' Intent to Stay in Hospital: A Comparison Across Five Occupational Categories", *International Journal for Quality in Health Care*, Vol. 26, No. 2, pp. 158-166, April, http://dx.doi.org/10.1093/intqhc/mzu006.

Hussein, S., M. Stevens and J. Manthorpe (2011), "What Drives the Recruitment of Migrant Workers to Work in Social Care in England?, *Social Policy and Society*, Vol. 10, pp. 285-298.

Hysong, S.J., R.G. Best and F.I. Moore (2007), "Are We Under-utilizing the Talents of Primary Care Personnel? A Job Analytic Examination", Implement Science, Vol. 2:10, March.

Klegeris, A. and H. Hurren (2011), "Impact of Problem-based Learning in a Large Classroom Setting: Student Perception and Problem-solving Skills", *Advances in Physiology Education*, Vol. 35, pp. 408-415.

Lizarondo, L. et al. (2010), "Allied Health Assistants and What They Do: A Systematic Review of the Literature", *Journal of Multidisciplinary Healthcare*, Vol. 19, No. 3, pp. 143-153, August.

Mache, S. et al. (2012), "Doctors' Working Conditions in Emergency Care Units in Germany: A Real-time Assessment", *Emergency Medicine Journal*, Vol. 29, No. 12, e1, December.

National Audit Office (2009), *Skills for Health. A Review by the National Audit Office*, NAO, London.

OECD (2015), *Health at a Glance 2015: OECD Indicators*, OECD Publishing, Paris, http://dx.doi.org/10.1787/health_glance-2015-en.

OECD (2014), *OECD Reviews of Health Care Quality: Italy 2014: Raising Standards*, OECD Publishing, Paris, http://dx.doi.org/10.1787/9789264225428-en.

OECD (2013), *OECD Skills Outlook 2013: First Results from the Survey of Adult Skills*, OECD Publishing, Paris, http://dx.doi.org/10.1787/9789264204256-en.

Ono, T., G. Lafortune and M. Schoenstein (2013), "Health Workforce Planning in OECD Countries: A Review of 26 Projection Models from 18 Countries", *OECD Health Working Papers*, No. 62, OECD Publishing, Paris, http://dx.doi.org/10.1787/5k44t787zcwb-en.

Quintini, G. (2011a), "Over-Qualified or Under-Skilled: A Review of Existing Literature", *OECD Social, Employment and Migration Working Papers*, No. 121, OECD Publishing, Paris, http://dx.doi.org/10.1787/5kg58j9d7b6d-en.

Quintini, G. (2011b), "Right for the Job: Over-Qualified or Under-Skilled?", *OECD Social, Employment and Migration Working Papers*, No. 120, OECD Publishing, Paris, http://dx.doi.org/10.1787/5kg59fcz3tkd-en.

Skochelak, S. (2010), "A Century of Progress in Medical Education: What About the Next 10 Years?", *Academic Medicine*, Vol. 85, pp. 197-200.

Van Bogaert, P. et al. (2013a), "Nursing Unit Teams Matter: Impact of Unit-level Nurse Practice Environment, Nurse Work Characteristics, and Burnout on Nurse Reported Job Outcomes, and Quality of Care, and Patient Adverse Events-A Cross-sectional Survey", *International Journal of Nursing Studies*, ePub 2013 December 30.

Van Bogaert, P. et al. (2013b), "The Relationship Between Nurse Practice Environment, Nurse Work Characteristics, Burnout and Job Outcome and Quality of Nursing Care: A Cross-sectional Survey", *International Journal of Nursing Studies*, Vol. 50, No. 12, pp. 1667-1677, December.

Van Riemsdijk, M. (2013), "Everyday Geopolitics, the Valuation of Labour and the Socio-Political Hierarchies of Skill: Polish Nurses in Norway", *Journal of Ethnic and Migration Studies*, Vol. 39, No. 3, pp. 373-390.

ORGANISATION FOR ECONOMIC CO-OPERATION AND DEVELOPMENT

The OECD is a unique forum where governments work together to address the economic, social and environmental challenges of globalisation. The OECD is also at the forefront of efforts to understand and to help governments respond to new developments and concerns, such as corporate governance, the information economy and the challenges of an ageing population. The Organisation provides a setting where governments can compare policy experiences, seek answers to common problems, identify good practice and work to co-ordinate domestic and international policies.

The OECD member countries are: Australia, Austria, Belgium, Canada, Chile, the Czech Republic, Denmark, Estonia, Finland, France, Germany, Greece, Hungary, Iceland, Ireland, Israel, Italy, Japan, Korea, Luxembourg, Mexico, the Netherlands, New Zealand, Norway, Poland, Portugal, the Slovak Republic, Slovenia, Spain, Sweden, Switzerland, Turkey, the United Kingdom and the United States. The European Union takes part in the work of the OECD.

OECD Publishing disseminates widely the results of the Organisation's statistics gathering and research on economic, social and environmental issues, as well as the conventions, guidelines and standards agreed by its members.

OECD PUBLISHING, 2, rue André-Pascal, 75775 PARIS CEDEX 16
(81 2015 18 1 P) ISBN 978-92-64-23950-0 – 2016

www.ingramcontent.com/pod-product-compliance
Ingram Content Group UK Ltd.
Pitfield, Milton Keynes, MK11 3LW, UK
UKHW051502290926
15471UKWH00008B/1357

9 789264 239500